A Duck Out of Water

Mum, dementia and care home life

Helen Johns

Published by New Generation Publishing in 2023

Copyright © 2023 Helen Johns

Front cover design by Cyan Rose Design *https://www.cyanrosedesign.co.uk*

First Edition

ISBNs:

Paperback: 978-1-80369-685-0
eBook: 978-1-80369-686-7

www.newgeneration-publishing.com

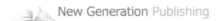

New Generation Publishing

Dedication

For Ian and The Lovely Rita – my fellow Musketeers.

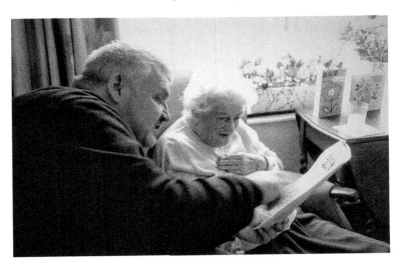

'Home isn't a place, it's a feeling' -
Cecelia Ahern, Love, Rosie

*****

'Rules for happiness: something to do, someone to love,
something to hope for.'
— Immanuel Kant

Acknowledgements

My thanks go …

To those who helped me bring this book to life. Linda, who read the very first draft of Part 1 and gently made suggestions that helped me on my way. Debbie, who had the dubious pleasure of reading my next attempt and made those sound observations that had me scuttling back to my laptop. Anne and Lorna, who in very different ways helped me push, pull and cajole my sentences into something resembling a coherent story. And to Julie and Aileen, who made sure I hadn't just made the whole thing up!

To Jenny Williams, for her editing skills to bring everything into shape and Cyan Fullbrook who designed the book cover which is a beautiful representation of our duck out of water.

To Michael Heppell, who brought me together with my fantastic friends and accountability groups in the Write That Book Masterclass and Team 17. Your encouragement kept me going when I wanted to hide and wondered why on earth I was doing this.

To my long-standing, long-suffering friends, who endured years (and I mean years) of me turning every conversation into an opportunity to rant about dementia, care homes and arguments about social care. I know that, for a while, I turned a tiny bit deranged.

To my wise and wonderful husband Ian, who was by my side every step of the way. Not only for the writing of the book, but for the years when Mum, dementia and care home life engulfed our world. You know this story because you saw everything and felt it too. You accepted this almighty challenge with good grace, patience and love for me and Mum. Thank you for every time you rescued my fragile soul and helped me carry on.

Finally, to my beautiful mum – the duck out of water. You have taught me so much in the past ten years and without your guidance – often cutting through the dementia – I would have been lost. Your beautiful smile will stay with me forever.

Letter to the Reader

Dear Reader,

When I decided to write this book, I had a choice to make. Should I simply tell the story of the heartache of dementia and gloss over the other hardships we faced as a family? After some agonising, I felt that this would merely tell half the story and decided that, if I was going to honour Mum properly, I had to be honest about our whole experience. This is a 'mother and daughter' story; after years of living with fear and worry, I needed to get brave and share my truth.

This book was created by referring to a collection of scraps of paper, loose sheets, printed notes, minutes of meetings and multiple notebooks that tell a story of my mum's experience of living with dementia in a care home.

Conversations are as I remember them, and scenes described as best as my memory will allow – but nothing in this book is 'make-believe.' Sometimes I have used the exact words that Mum said – I know, because I made a note of them at the time – sometimes mispronounced or jumbled.

It was difficult to relive some events as they reminded me of her pain, but I did so to illustrate the reality of her life at that time. I have included my observations, thoughts, feelings and opinions about the events, people and organisations we encountered. They are just that – my views on our experience; others may have a different experience and perspective.

I have also had to confront what I did, or didn't, do for Mum at various points. I have questioned my actions hundreds of times. I am not a perfect daughter – I just did what I thought was right at the time. The benefit of hindsight is great, and, in my shoes, you may or may not have done the same.

Inevitably, there are some aspects I describe that are deeply personal issues – particularly around Mum's incontinence. Some may feel that this is an invasion of her privacy, and to a certain extent it is. However, anything I chose to include was purely to illustrate a realistic picture of her declining health and what was done to try to improve it.

I have changed the names and sometimes the gender of individuals, except where I have specific permission from family and friends to use their real names. This is a personal memoir, and I did not want to identify any person that we encountered in their professional capacity.

Throughout the book, I use the term 'resident' to describe people who live in a care home. It was certainly not my intention to generalise about the diverse individuals who became my friends and that I grew to love – but, for ease of reading, I have used the term to distinguish between them and others in the story.

To those who were part of the story and showed Mum love, respect, warmth and kindness – thank you from the bottom of my heart. You know who you are. You made Mum happy; you retained her dignity and her sense of being herself. In doing so, you kept me sane, gave me hope and helped me find the strength to keep going when I wanted to give up.

To those who are surprised, angered or hurt by the things they read – my intention was then, and still is now, simply to be heard and helped to improve Mum's care. I regret that I wasn't always able to communicate my messages better, and that the time and place weren't right for a change in the culture of care, BUT I do not regret that I kept trying on Mum's behalf. I'm not sorry that I kept thinking of her feelings and asking everyone involved to do the same.

To any informal carers or relatives who are embarking on their own path, I hope that, in sharing our story, you gain a further insight and knowledge into dementia care. I hope it gives you the courage to keep going, even when you do not want to. From my own experience, I know there will be times when you doubt yourself, question your expectations, or be persuaded to do the same by others. I hope this book helps you understand that you are not alone and that – when your focus is on protecting your loved one's wellbeing – you are doing the right thing. Perhaps our story is one that you are already familiar with and, if so, I wish you strength and resilience on your journey.

Most importantly, this book does not provide medical advice or treatment options, or indeed recommend any course of action around social care. However, it does describe what worked *for us*.

Mum's dementia changed my life both personally and professionally. I have now seen the care system from both sides. If you are a care home professional and think 'not in my home', I urge you to take another look. The events I describe are ordinary happenings and I have seen similar in care homes other than my mum's. People, like those who feature in this book, with their heart-warming acts of kindness, are all around us. So, too, are those who make care home life dull, miserable and heartbreaking. I'm not talking about blatant cruelty or neglect; my mum's story doesn't include any of those horrors. It is a damage that is more subtle. Those staff who, for whatever reason, fail to see the important things that make us human. They are the ones who do, or say, seemingly insignificant things that erode a person's sense of self. You may not notice it at first, but to someone living with dementia, each little infringement will be felt deeply. Look closer, take action, challenge where you can, and make a change.

While I was writing our story, Covid-19 erupted and swept across the world. During that time, care homes were under enormous pressure and care staff worked hard at protecting our loved ones. I do not underestimate the role they have played in keeping vulnerable people safe and the burden they have carried – at that time and since. *Thank you.*

It was my sincere intention to do something positive by writing this book and being honest about our experience. It is only by having gone through this experience that I have developed any expertise. I didn't set out to absorb myself in the world of dementia or care homes but dementia chose Mum and so by default, chose me. Now I am glad it did. Dementia has taught me so much about loving, living and learning – it has changed me for ever.

Whatever route your own path takes you – I wish you the very best.

Helen

x

Contents

Part 1

A Duck Out of Water

Chapter 1

'How did I get here?':
From Home to Care Home

Leading up to December 2012

In November 2012 my lovely mother, Rita, was diagnosed with vascular dementia and, less than two months later, she moved into a care home. Many people who have that same diagnosis live happily in their own homes, for years. So how did my mother end up living in a care home so quickly?

Mum was a bit of a 'creaking gate' as we were growing up. From the bunions she had in the 1970s to the migraines that caused her to lie in a darkened room for hours on end – she endured a lot. She also suffered with low mood, anxiety and depression. At one point this led to her having panic attacks and she sometimes struggled to leave the house. There always seemed to be something ailing her but, somehow, she muddled along. Mum's troubles lurked in the background, but they didn't stop her from being a warm, loving wife and a caring mother to her three daughters. Of course, her girls worried about her, but we saw how she rallied from every setback. It was the way Mum was.

As each of us flew the nest we became preoccupied with our own lives, but we stayed in touch and visited regularly. Aileen, my oldest sister, lived close to Mum and when Ian, the first grandson arrived, Grandma Rita helped with childcare so that Aileen could continue working. Barbara, my middle sister, moved to Australia in the 1980s but was probably most attuned to Mum's health. They exchanged long newsy letters or phone calls and had a strong bond, despite the distance. I, the youngest, also lived near Mum but focussed on my career and social life and didn't make as much time for her as I could have. Of course, I loved her, but I didn't pay close attention to her day-to-day life.

Our dad, Leo, died unexpectedly in 2001, but Mum continued to live in our modest family home. When she became less mobile, she needed the help of carers, but otherwise, she managed well. In 2002 she was diagnosed with Type 2 diabetes, but our treat-loving mother did not let that stand in the way of eating exactly what she wanted. She ignored suggestions of lifestyle changes and rumbled along – mostly without incident.

A few years on, after a couple of falls and new health issues, all three daughters suggested it was time for a move to somewhere smaller and more secure. We found a council-run sheltered accommodation complex only two streets away from Aileen's house. Initially, Mum was reluctant, but on seeing the bright, airy one-bedroom flat, she changed her mind. In 2004 she moved to what became her cosy, comfortable haven, and lived there contentedly for the next eight years. She spent her time pottering around the flat, sometimes dabbling in her old hobbies of sketching, painting, reading, and writing poetry. She also took up a new and prolific hobby – catalogue shopping – the results of which frustrated me to death.

It all changed for me around 2006. As Mum got older and frailer, I wanted to take care of her and started to appreciate the sweet lady who had brought us up so well. She had lots of hospital appointments and often needed an escort to drive her there and help her navigate the vast modern buildings. I ran my own business and had more flexibility than Aileen did, so I took up the role. Seeing her so frequently created a stronger bond between us. Her vulnerability touched me, but the changes I saw in her seemed to be the usual signs of getting older and I accepted them. We didn't hit any real problems until Mum's memory rapidly declined and that triggered the return of those long-standing anxieties. Her problems seemed to escalate so quickly. Yet, when I look back, there were signs of what was looming much earlier.

*****

For as long as I can remember, Mum was forgetful, and we were used to her misplacing various items. As she got older, she lost more things, more often, but I saw it as simply part of ageing. I would roll my eyes and sigh as I joined in another search of the flat for her purse or her keys.

Unconnected, or so I thought, she was referred to a local memory clinic as she started to struggle with word-finding. In the middle of a conversation, she would hesitate and say, 'What's the word I want? I can't find it. I can see it in my mind but can't find it.'

It frustrated Mum but, again, I assumed it was part of growing older and that the psychiatrist at the clinic was keeping an eye on it. Mum had taken several memory tests, but the results didn't alarm or alert me to a bigger problem looming.

We were all about to encounter something different.

My first experience of Mum saying something odd came out of the blue. One day, while visiting her, I made us both a cup of tea in the tiny kitchen of her flat. The kitchen led directly from the living room where Mum sat chatting away through the open doorway. Out of nowhere I heard her say, 'Where's Leo?' I stopped short and popped my head through the doorway.

'D'you mean Dad, Mam?'

I thought she'd mixed up family members' names and meant someone else. Someone alive.

'Yes – where is he?'

I put down the cup I was holding and joined her on the two-seater sofa.

'Mam,' I said, hesitating as I thought of how to phrase the next bit as gently as I could. 'Dad died a few years ago. Don't you remember?'

'Oh yes!' she replied, and seemed to snap back to the present time. She reacted as if she'd merely forgotten what day of the week it was and didn't appear disturbed by the news. Relieved, I went back to the kitchen, made the drinks, and moved on. She had remembered quickly and didn't mention him again that day, so I didn't think any more of it.

Similar things started to happen but, at first, there were lengthy periods between each incident. I mentioned them to Aileen but, as they were sporadic, we didn't suspect anything serious. If anything, we became preoccupied with (or perhaps distracted by) a physical condition that we thought was the source of her intermittent confusion.

Among Mum's other ailments were her various 'toilet troubles' – including recurring Urinary Tract Infections (UTIs). These made her uncomfortable and somewhat incontinent but, like everything else, she dealt with them. However, they became more frequent over the years and together my sister and I worked out that they coincided with the episodes of confusion. I was baffled, so scoured the internet for information and learned that diabetes could cause a weaker immune system which, in turn, could make people more prone to UTIs. I also learned that UTIs could cause sudden confusion (or delirium) in the elderly. I cobbled these bits of information together and thought I had our answer: *Mum's diabetes means that she has frequent UTIs, which in turn cause her confusion.*

Armed with that information, Aileen and I increased our vigilance and developed a well-honed routine for spotting signs of Mum having a UTI. If she said or did something that seemed odd, that would sound alarm bells and we would ask the District Nurse who visited Mum daily for insulin injections to take a urine sample. That inevitably resulted in a confirmed case of a UTI and a prescription for a course of antibiotics. A few days into the course, Mum's symptoms abated, and we breathed a sigh of relief. A period of normality followed but in a couple of months the cycle started again.

We knew the antibiotics worked but saw how Mum became more worried by each bout of confusion.

'Our Helen – that thing is starting again. I feel funny.' She knew something was wrong.

We needed a different approach that prevented the UTIs from occurring in the first place. More internet research and suggestions followed: adjustments to Mum's diet and encouraging her to drink more water. We were on it! We slavishly followed this regime for months but felt defeated when, despite our efforts, the UTIs returned, as did her confusion.

With each new infection, the depth of her confusion grew. As well as the questions about Dad, she now asked about our grandma and grandad who had both died in the 1970s. She started to talk about 'going home', despite being in the flat that she'd lived in for eight years. I didn't know where she meant but, thankfully, at that time, my prompts and reminders brought her back to the present. I had no idea what was going on but as Mum's six-monthly appointment for the memory clinic was due, I decided to speak to the psychiatrist about these episodes.

Check-up appointments usually took place in Mum's flat and involved careful manoeuvres on my part to give the psychiatrist an accurate picture of the situation without alarming Mum. That day was no different. As usual, the psychiatrist asked Mum how she was coping memory-wise, and she gave a polite and positive response. I didn't want to contradict her but tried subtly to suggest this might not be the whole story. My usual facial expressions, wide eyes or subtly shaking my head, felt disloyal to Mum, so this time I made an excuse to see the psychiatrist alone. I was ashamed of my dishonesty but needed to speak openly. In those snatched moments, I shared the worrying news of the frequent UTIs, confusion, and mishaps since the last appointment. I hoped for answers but, with limited time, I struggled to convey all the detail or to stress how worried I was about my lovely mother.

The psychiatrist reassured me that any infection in the body could cause delirium so I could assume that the UTI was the cause. *Good, I thought. I've got that. I'm doing the right thing in managing the UTIs. Keep going.* I relayed this to Aileen, and we continued our mission. Each day one of us checked in on Mum and we were relieved when there were no signs of confusion. I enthusiastically kept a tally of how many days since the last infection, but my optimism soon plummeted when a bewildered Mum reached out to one of us for help.

As the months passed, the confusion took on a new dimension. Mum was not only muddled but she was also afraid. She sensed something bad was happening to her and sought comfort in finding somewhere familiar. She became more preoccupied with getting 'back home' and my feeble reminders that she was already at home were starting to lose their impact. *Try logic*, I thought.

'Remember, Mam, this is your sofa, this is your china cabinet – all your things are in it. This must be where you live.'

She looked at each item as I pointed to them but was unconvinced. She scrunched up her eyes and said, 'Live here? No ... I'm not sure.' Then: 'How did I get here?'

Fed up with watching her suffer more with each UTI, I took Mum to her GP to discuss what we could do to break the cycle. He sympathised with our frustrations but suggested that this could be something more long-term. He didn't say the word 'dementia', but suddenly I knew what he meant. *God, I didn't even consider that!* I thought, embarrassed at my naivety. *Is that what she's got?* I had been so convinced it was all about the UTIs that I hadn't even thought of anything else. I hadn't linked all the elements: Mum's day-to-day forgetfulness, the difficulty with word-finding, the confusion about long-dead relatives and not recognising her own home. *They might all be part of the same problem.*

We left the GP surgery, and I was more uncertain than ever about what was happening to Mum. Months passed and each healthcare professional repeated their differing opinions. I grew desperate for a clear steer as to whether Mum's confusion was from the multiple UTIs or if she did have dementia. We were in limbo for what seemed like an age. The uncertainty eventually ended as her dementia progressed rapidly and a series of events occurred that left us in no doubt.

*****

My partner, Ian, and I were due to get married in September 2012. We had already been together for fifteen years but decided to go all out and have a small but 'proper' do. The venue was booked, preparations were in place and we all looked forward to a celebration. Barbara and her family were arriving from Australia – it would be a whole-family affair.

Three weeks before the wedding, disaster struck. Mum fell in her flat and broke her knee. She needed a short stay in hospital but while there she packed her bags daily and asked to go home. A nurse confirmed that she had another UTI, but I was sure that being in an unfamiliar environment unsettled her further. *We would all want to go home, wouldn't we?* On the day of the wedding, she was allowed out on 'day release' and I was thrilled to have her there in her stylish mother-of-the-bride outfit and being made a fuss of by friends and relatives. Days later, Barbara told me that she'd not really understood what was going on during the day and had become a little angry as a result. *Poor Mam, she usually loved a wedding!*

Two weeks later, the knee was healing so she was allowed home. Ian and I collected her from the hospital, stuffing our car with walking aids and other paraphernalia. The car looked like the wagon from the American sitcom *The Beverly Hillbillies*. Mum sat in the back squashed between her belongings but beamed as she was finally going home. She was thrilled and so were we – everything would be better once she was back at home.

That wasn't to be. Within days the stark reality hit as Mum displayed all the symptoms we'd seen before, but this time without any UTI. *This is it. It must be dementia,* I thought. I begged professionals to explain exactly what was happening. We needed a diagnosis. The term 'mild cognitive impairment' was used but I didn't know exactly what that meant. *Is that the start of dementia?* I understood the words but not what it meant *to us.* One afternoon, I argued with a Community Psychiatric Nurse (CPN) who questioned why I needed to know what 'it' was. Did it matter? Would it mean I treated her differently? I resented this and ruminated endlessly on our conversation. *How can a professional not understand that I need to know? Surely the correct diagnosis could help us consider what to do next.* For me, we had a simple question that needed answering. Did we need to prepare ourselves to manage Mum's UTIs, or did she have a progressive disease that was likely to have a permanent impact on her life?

We waited for a diagnosis. Meanwhile, Mum was suffering more, and we had daily proof of the turmoil she endured. She made phone calls to me or Aileen in the early hours of the morning, alerting us to another confused episode that frightened her. They seemed to follow a pattern: Mum would wake up in the middle of the night disorientated and call me to ask if I could take her home. I would gently remind her that she was a little disorientated because she had just woken up, that she was in the right place, not to worry, and we could sort things out in the morning. She would accept my explanation and go back to bed. My stomach was in knots almost every evening, but I was comforted knowing that she always called if she was scared.

I visited her daily now and usually arrived to find the result of the previous night's confusion. She often emptied the drawers in her bedroom and packed bags ready to leave. I'd reassure her that she was at home, and when she was ready, we returned each item back to the drawers – only to do the same again the day after.

One morning, I found a note she'd written in the middle of the previous night. It was addressed to whoever owned the flat she was in (believing it not to be hers). I winced as I read the polite note, in which she apologised for having slept on their bed. She explained that she was exhausted and had to lie down. I imagined her being riddled with worry about intruding in someone else's home, trying hard not to fall asleep but being so tired that she eventually gave in. *You poor thing,* I thought, as I popped the note into my handbag. I didn't want her to see it again and be frightened by what she'd written.

I never knew what would happen next.

Late one November afternoon, I found her sitting alone, in the dark. Usually, the TV or radio was playing – Mum said it gave her a 'bit of company' – but not that afternoon. She sat in the silence, staring into space.

'What's up, Mam?' I asked.

'I don't know.' She looked dazed

'Are you okay, though? Do you feel poorly?

'No ... I'm alright.'

'Why are you sitting in the dark?'

'I don't know.'

'Shall I put a light on?' I wanted to make everything normal again. 'Don't you want to watch something on the telly?'

'If you like,' she said.

That day, it didn't occur to her that sitting in the dark with no stimulation was a strange thing to do.

I noticed that her confusion got worse later in the day as it began to get dark. The urge to go home was strongest then; I now know this as 'sundowning,' a common symptom of dementia. Back then, I simply witnessed her becoming agitated when faced with the prospect of staying in this flat that she didn't recognise as her home.

On another visit, I discovered this feeling was getting worse for Mum. As I arrived at the building, the warden of the flats beckoned me to her office.

'Can I have a quick word?'

'Yes – is everything okay? I knew it wasn't from the concerned look fixed on her face.

'Your mam has been disturbing some of the other residents in the middle of the night.'

'Oh God! What happened?'

'Well, she knocked on Jimmy's and on Mary's door. They told me this morning. She said that she was lost, had they seen her mother and could they help her get home.'

My heart hit the floor like a stone.

'That's terrible,' I said. 'Poor Mam, she must have been terrified to leave the flat at night. It's not like her. Can you tell them I'm really sorry?'

'I just thought I'd let you know. I have to think about the other residents.'

Inside, I thought, *this is getting worse – it's now affecting other people.* I hoped that she wouldn't say any more. 'I'm really sorry. I'll try and sort it out. I'll see how she is today.'

I headed for the stairs towards Mum's flat, knowing full well that I had no idea how to sort this out. Our problems were coming thick and fast.

The carers told us of various mishaps they'd encountered on their visits. They called four times a day, but now Mum was afraid whenever she was alone. Aileen and I took turns sitting with her between the teatime carer leaving and the bedtime carer arriving.

We tried to soothe her by watching TV together, chatting, reading magazines or playing cards. Sometimes we did little household tasks together and that seemed to help too. She needed companionship and repeated reassurances. Sometimes it worked, but it became increasingly difficult to relieve her anxiety.

In the November, in yet another meeting with professionals, I managed to tease out a vague verbal diagnosis of dementia but, even then, I felt I was prising information from them. I couldn't understand the problem with giving a clear diagnosis. Practical information was thin on the ground, we didn't know enough about dementia, and so we frantically dealt with each problem as it arose. We were simply fighting fires. Mum had more episodes of anxiety and the gaps between them got shorter. We were rapidly losing our ability to pacify her for even a short while.

A feeling of impending doom hung upon me, and I tried to understand what might lie ahead for Mum. I had more unanswered questions. *How will she change? What care will she need? How will this change her life – and ours too?* The worries came and went all day long. I knew this wasn't solely a clinical matter – it was much more now. Our lives were about to change. A few short weeks after that diagnosis, we reached a crisis point – our saddest day.

Chapter 2

'Our saddest day ever': Tough Decisions

December 2012

On a bright, sunny Saturday morning early in December, things came to a head. Ian and I were out shopping when my mobile phone rang and one of Mum's neighbours told me that he had found her in tears at the foyer of the building. She told him that she was lost and needed her mother. *Oh my God,* I thought, the now-familiar knotted feeling returning to my stomach. *This is bad. Why didn't she ring me?* I'd always felt reassured that if she was scared, she'd contact me or Aileen. Thankfully, the neighbour had comforted her enough to persuade her to come back to her own flat and had found my number perched next to the phone.

'I'll be there in fifteen minutes,' I said, and we swung into the emergency response mode that had become part of our lives over the last few months.

Mum looked startled as I walked into the living room, and continued to stare wide eyed as I stood beside her chair. Usually, she calmed down when one of us arrived, but this time seemed different. I crouched down beside her and took her hand.

'Hi, Mam. What's up?'

Her face crumpled and tears streamed down her face.

'Oh, don't cry, Mam. You're okay – we'll stay here with you.'

'I just want to go home,' she sobbed.

'You *are* at home, Mam.' I doubted that my usual orientation tactics would work now but, caught off guard, I tried them.

'Look – it's that lovely armchair you bought,' I said, stroking the arm of the chair. She looked at it blankly. I tried again. 'Look, there's your china cabinet with all your things in it.' I scanned the room looking for something else that I thought she might remember. 'This is the lovely green carpet you bought.' I hoped she'd recognise the dark green colour that she'd fallen in love with and insisted on buying a few years earlier. Still nothing.

'Please. Just take me home,' she pleaded through her tears.

My stomach clenched again as I listened to my poor mum, begging me to take her somewhere that she thought of as home. *Where is this mystery home she wants? Does she want to be back at the house we grew up in?* I simply didn't know.

'I'm sorry, Mam, but you *are* home.'

I clung to a tiny bit of hope that this time my words would snap her back to reality, that she'd see her cosy flat and feel calm. Not today. The usual ways to reassure her had become less and less effective as each month passed, and today they were useless.

'Come on,' she said, 'let's go.' More insistent this time. Stupidly, I kept trying to reason with her. Sitting bolt upright, she clenched her fists and shouted. 'We have to leave! This is not our place – we have to go!' She was convinced that we were intruding in someone else's flat.

'How about a cup of tea before we go, then?' Ian pitched in, trying to buy time in the hope that it gave us a chance to calm things down. It didn't work one bit.

'No! Do – not – touch – *anything!*' she bellowed, emphasising each word. 'This is not our house, and we must not touch anything. We are good people.' Ian stood rooted to the spot, and patiently took the earbashing.

Within moments, she broke into more sobs. I tried to hold her hand, but she brushed me away. Still crouched beside her chair, I looked up towards Ian who I could see felt as helpless as I did. With no other choice, we knew we had to wait this out and meanwhile search for the words that would break through Mum's distress. Her confusion lasted for hours.

By late afternoon, Aileen and her husband, Alan, arrived. I hoped that fresh faces and voices would make a difference, but nothing worked. Worse still, our diabetic mum was refusing food. Low blood sugar, confusion, fear and anger were not a good recipe at this stage. I hoped that she would eventually feel sleepy and wake up having forgotten her distress. Not a chance. She was so agitated that she maintained a laser-like focus on the imminent trouble that she felt she was in. We were all out of ideas.

In desperation, Aileen contacted the out-of-hours GP who came and checked Mum over. She stated firmly that Mum was too distressed to be left alone and needed to go to the hospital as an emergency admission. We packed a bag and agreed that Aileen and Alan would take her. As they left, Mum seemed calmed by the fact that she was off to hospital, but I knew she didn't understand the full picture. She wouldn't have realised that she had to stay there. It felt like we were having her committed and taken away. My head knew that she needed to be somewhere safe, but my heart felt that I had let her down.

The previous six hours had been traumatic for everyone and, as I locked the door of the flat, I thought gloomily, *this is our saddest day ever.* I was emotionally drained, but my mind still raced on. *What will we do now? What's the next step?* It had reached the point where we, as a family, were unable to help Mum on our own.

Ian and I were due to go to a concert that evening but I felt frazzled and in no mood to be entertained. Ian reasoned that, as Mum was safe and looked after for the time being, a night out might distract me from my worries. If not, we could come straight back home. It felt wrong but I agreed. I sat in the concert hall listening to the music with tears rolling down my cheeks. My body was in the room, but my mind was with her. *Poor Mam. What can I do to help you?*

The following day, a new round of hospital visits began. A depressing feeling of déjà vu weighed heavy on me as I trudged back to the same hospital where Mum had stayed after her fall in the September. Aileen worked full time, so visited when she could, but for me it was like Groundhog Day. Every day – and sometimes twice a day – I'd arrive to find Mum looking lost and lonely. Invariably, one of the nurses would tell me she had packed and repacked her bag all day. I knew that she felt out of place in the hospital, with its strange sounds and unfamiliar faces. The ward was filled with people in different states of memory decline. I'm sure the sight of those vulnerable people unnerved Mum, as some wailed for help and others shouted out their frustration. This was my first experience of other people with dementia too and I was unsettled at seeing Mum looking so small and vulnerable among them. *I get it, Mam – for two pins I'd pack your bags myself and 'spring' you from here*, I thought protectively.

As if she didn't have enough to cope with, a new problem emerged: constipation. Mum's range of toilet troubles were now three-fold. Staving off those UTIs, her increasing incontinence, and now being bunged up at the other end. She panicked when in any toilet areas and every trip to the bathroom was an ordeal for her. She was beset with worries and the nursing staff were unable to reassure her for long. The NHS is a brilliant service, filled with hardworking and caring professionals, but the reality is that hospitals are not set up for caring for those living with dementia. Busy staff, understandably, focus on medical needs, and unfortunately the ever-present reassurance that people living with dementia need cannot be given.

Mum was in hospital for three weeks but, soon after admission, all the professionals concluded that she could no longer live alone and needed 24-hour care. Having lived through the previous months of Mum's distress, we agreed with their decision and knew we needed to find a suitable care home. Almost immediately, I felt pressurised by a social worker who cautioned me that I'd need to get a move on as hospitals didn't like people 'bed blocking.' *Bed blocking? I thought. She's only been there a few days.* I was catapulted into a high-speed care home search in which Aileen and I frantically worked through a list of care home names, shortlisting those we wanted to visit.

We knew we needed to get this next move right for our fragile, nervy mother. She had a long history of visiting our grandma who had been in and out of hospitals in the 1960s and early '70s. Grandma was described as being 'bad with her nerves', which in today's terms would be known as having mental health illnesses. As children, we were shielded from the detail, but I knew that Mum had incredibly sad memories associated with that time and the institutions that Grandma stayed in. Anything clinical was no good for Mum; we needed something more homely. It wasn't about whether there was posh wallpaper or plush carpets, but we needed to find somewhere cosy that suited Mum's personality and didn't trigger those memories. Our wish list was modest: a cosy bedroom with a private bathroom, a homely communal lounge for meeting companions and a garden so she could enjoy the outdoor space. The home needed to be within easy driving distance for both of us so that we could visit often.

After a few unsuccessful viewings, we visited a care home that Aileen's colleague had suggested. The deputy manager guided us through the building, showing us what was on offer. As we walked through the neutral-coloured corridors and homely lounges filled with muted soft furnishings, there seemed to be a pleasant atmosphere. She took us to a bright, spacious bedroom on the first floor with a large window that overlooked the garden. My heart leapt at this prospect as I gazed out towards the lawn. *Mam will love being able to see a garden,* I thought. I scanned the room and imagined her recliner chair and a few ornaments in there. *We can make this lovely.*

The deputy manager explained more about the home and their approach. They welcomed residents and their families and wanted everyone to feel reassured throughout their stay. 'We never want you to leave here with a heavy heart,' she said. I beamed at this lovely, touching sentiment and it sealed the deal for me. *Mam will be happy here, and they care about relatives as well.*

Aileen was convinced that the room number, 25, was a good omen. In the car park she told me of the connections:

'Our first family home was number 25, Grandad and Grandma lived in number 25, and we live at number 25. It's a good sign – she will be happy here.'

'Shall we go for it, then?' I asked her.

'Yes – I think this is the one, Helen.'

'Let's do it, then.'

For the first time in months, I felt optimistic believing that we might be able to help Mum move on from the worries she'd had when living independently. She could live in this safe and comfortable place where there was 24-hour care available. I breathed a sigh of relief and arranged for her to move in within a week. I was convinced that it offered all the things she needed. The question of exactly how that home catered for Mum's *emotional wellbeing* did not arise until later.

Chapter 3
'Happy New Year!': A Fresh Start for All of Us
January 2013

On the last day of 2012, Mum moved into the care home that became her home for almost seven years. That morning, Aileen and I brought her clothes and a few small items from the flat to make her bedroom cosier and more familiar. I made the bed with the beige paisley-print duvet cover that Mum loved so much. A bunch of roses stood in Grandma's old vase on the chest of drawers, and I placed framed photos on the windowsill. We were allowed to bring Mum's comfy recliner bed and chair which was due to arrive at the end of the week. Later that afternoon, I collected Mum from the hospital, and spent the next few hours settling her into her new abode. We walked the corridors and checked out each of the communal spaces. By early evening, Mum was tired, so I kissed her goodbye and promised to return the next morning after her breakfast.

It was New Year's Eve, but I didn't care about celebrations that year. I wanted the morning to come quickly so that I could see Mum again and check that she was okay.

The next day, I awoke early but distracted myself with chores until what I thought was a reasonable time to leave. Ian reminded me that I'd need to give staff a chance to get Mum up and dressed, and for her to have breakfast, before I arrived – but the wait was torture. As we drove to the home, my stomach did somersaults, and I willed myself to think positive thoughts. When we got to the front door, I was so nervous that I couldn't work out which of the keypad buttons was the doorbell, so I knocked on the door and peered through the glass. Thankfully, I caught the attention of a passing carer who let us in and showed us to the lift. As we arrived at the first floor, we were greeted by another carer who said Mum had had a good night's sleep. *Thank God. She's finally got some peace,* I thought, as I hurried to her room. Mum was sat in a chair at the far side of the room, absorbed in a magazine.

'Happy New Year, Mam!' I said, as I bounded in, rushing to hug her. I wrapped my arms around her big cuddly tummy and nuzzled in.

'Happy New Year to you too,' she replied, smiling widely. I was sure she didn't know the date, but she was always polite enough to return any greeting.

'You look great, Mam.' I was chuffed to see her pure-white curly hair looking properly styled and her clothes looking neat.

'Isn't this a lovely cosy room? Do you like it?' I was over-keen for her approval so I asked too many questions.

'Yes – it's nice', was all she said, but as she was smiling for the first time in a long while, that was enough for me.

I rambled on, pointing to the few items that we had brought from the flat, thinking she'd find comfort in the familiar possessions. She smiled and nodded as I sat on the floor close to her chair, hugging her knees every few minutes. I could hardly believe we had got her out of the hospital as I thought to myself, *she'll be at home here.*

The building had a quiet air about it which I assumed was because of the bank holiday. There weren't many people around, but I introduced myself to the carers I saw – different to those I'd met the day before but still pleasant and friendly. In Mum's bedroom,

I perched on the bed and the three of us chatted away. I couldn't contain my enthusiasm for this brilliant new abode, and I raved about each thing I saw as if it was a brand-new invention: 'Look, Mam, this is your private bathroom.' I wanted her to know that everything was okay now.

At around 12.30 pm one of the carers knocked on the door, even though it was open. I was impressed by the act of courtesy.

'It's time for lunch now, Rita,' she said cheerfully.

Mum looked to me for her answer.

'Yes, Mam, you can have some lunch here for free. Isn't that lovely?' Overemphasising yet another benefit.

'Okay then – if you don't mind,' she said, smiling timidly at the warm middle-aged woman. She heaved herself up from the chair and started towards the door. Relieved at how well this was going, we took it as our cue to go. I gave her another kiss, and Ian and I waved goodbye as we made our way to the lift, both of us beaming.

Back in the car, I turned to Ian. 'We've done it. At last, she's safe.'

'I know – it looks lovely,' he said.

'God, I feel I can breathe again.' I put my head in my hands – this time with relief. 'Did you think she looked happy?' I looked to him for confirmation.

'Yes – she seemed fine. Don't worry.'

'The best thing is, they'll be able to look after her if she's scared in between our visits.'

'They will. They'll know what to do.'

'I know – this is a good new start for her.'

'And for us,' Ian reminded me.

As he drove us away, I leaned back into the seat, stretching out fully and feeling relieved. We had a safety net now. No more worrying about where she was and what she was doing.

*****

My mum has dementia, and she lives in a care home. I kept saying these words in my head but the whole thing seemed unreal. I never dreamt that this would happen, so I didn't know what to expect or how to behave. Each new day in the home was an encounter with the unknown and all of it meant I had questions: *Where should I put Mum's dirty laundry? Can she have prunes for breakfast? Who deals with the medication? Who do I talk to about Mum's care?* I learned that on each floor there was a senior carer ('the Senior') and that they were my point of contact on a day-to-day basis. My head swam with a sea of questions about the minutiae of Mum's life, but I tried to curb the urge to ask everything at once.

My first priority was making Mum comfortable, and I set about trying to create a mini version of her flat so that she'd feel at home. Her recliner chair, comfortable bed and TV arrived that first week and I brought more clothes, ornaments and trinkets on each of my daily visits. The magnolia walls were light but bland, so I hung a couple of her own paintings alongside photos of family members. I brought books and magazines and a small CD player so she could have music around her. When I was done, I took photos on my phone and sent them to my sisters who congratulated me on the job. It looked cosy and Mum seemed comfortable, so I prayed that it helped her settle in.

Little did she know that, behind the scenes, I was dismantling her precious flat and was trying to find homes for the many items that simply would not fit into her cosy little bedroom.

*****

Mum and I have always been different in lots of respects. I like order, routine and organised cupboards – Mum was a bit of a hoarder. Not in a severe way but bad enough to have cupboards stuffed with possessions gathered over the years. Well before dementia appeared, she frequently lost things because of the sheer amount of 'stuff' she'd accumulated. Of course, her love of catalogue shopping compounded the problem and sometimes caused arguments between us.

For several years I had tried to cajole, persuade and, to an extent, bully her into letting some of her countless possessions go. However, my mother was steadfast and ignored my rationale for decluttering in any way. She applied the same value to a tattered old magazine from three years earlier as she did to a much-loved heirloom from Grandma. She wanted to keep it all, and that often resulted in a battle of wills: Mum would remain stubborn about the importance of a used postage stamp, and I would resent it. I thought she was maddening and ridiculous. She thought I was cold-hearted for not valuing things as she did.

Despite those arguments, I always tried again when we both felt calmer, and the prickly sorting routine continued. Years later, our persistence paid off. I used the photos, postcards and trinkets rescued from the overstuffed cupboards to create an impressive memory book for Mum. We used this to reminisce together for years to come and her carers were fascinated by its contents. I was glad that we had saved those precious items.

However, back in those first two weeks of January 2013, I was filled with dread at the prospect of getting rid of this suddenly redundant hoard. Aileen and I worked in shifts at clearing rooms and exchanged texts when either of us got stuck. Everything that Mum needed now was with her at the care home. Precious photos and cards were stored at my house, along with a couple of cherished pieces of furniture. The remaining items were the problem, and the sheer volume was overwhelming.

Ironically, I agonised over items that I'd previously thought of as worthless, and felt a deep sense of disloyalty as I packed another box for the charity shop. I knew on an intellectual level that this was the right thing to do, but emotionally it felt bad to discard the things that had made our mother so happy. Karma was in place. The daughter who had been Mum's clutter police for years now had the onerous task of making tough decisions about the future of all this stuff. She would have shot me and Aileen stone-dead if she had known that her possessions were being given away to charity shops, friends of friends, and anyone else who was willing to take the numerous surplus items.

On the last day at the flat, after everything had gone, I looked around at the empty rooms and reflected on how happy Mum had been in this little haven, surrounded by her 'stuff'. I cringed briefly at the thought of where it had all gone, but then brushed the uncomfortable feeling aside – it was time for a new chapter. Over the years, whenever new residents arrived at the care home, I always wondered whether their families were going through the same angst.

*****

Back at the care home, I took on a new mission: getting Mum's life organised. Care homes often ask relatives to label clothes in order to make sure that laundry is returned to the right person, but I took labelling to a whole new level. In her new bedroom, I made labels for every drawer so that she knew the contents of each one. I labelled the doors that led to the hall and the bathroom, so that she knew which was which. The TV remote control had her name on it, in case it was mistakenly taken out of the room. Walking frames, handbags, shoes ... you name it, it had a label on it.

I also love a gadget or tool and, over the coming years, I continued to buy or create more props to make Mum's life easier or to help the carers. I'm not a psychologist but I'm sure that what I was trying to do was to impose order into a world that was uncertain and unfamiliar for both of us. I thought that by keeping everything labelled and organised, I had a chance of keeping her orientated and happy. I was a novice at this care home malarkey, and I didn't realise that it would take so much more.

Chapter 4

'This is me!': Getting to Know Mum

January 2013

I wanted the care team in Mum's new home to get to know her. Not the medical information, which was available from her GP records, but other important things that made her feel comfortable and secure. After years of coordinating Mum's care, I knew that not everything was automatically included in care plans. For example, Mum didn't like the bitter taste of her pills so she preferred to take them with milk rather than water. Within the first week, I shared this information with the Senior on duty, who nodded but didn't make a note of it. *Okay*, I thought, *they know what they're doing*. I hoped that she'd remember and pass it on to other carers later.

I also wanted them to know about her personality and what she enjoyed doing during the day. As Mum wouldn't be able to explain things fully, I thought it was down to us to give them as much information as we knew. During the previous months of turmoil, we had been able to ease her anxiety by keeping her occupied. I thought that if carers encouraged her to do things she enjoyed, she might feel settled there.

I produced a summary of Mum's history on an A4 sheet and made a few copies. As well as listing the names of close family members, I made sure I included information about her personality: her friendly but timid ways, her gentle and loving disposition and her brilliant sense of humour. I noted down that she believed in God and had been a regular churchgoer. I wrote about her creative nature and mentioned that anything related to art, birds, flowers and plants interested her. I thought it was particularly important for them to know that she wrote poems and letters throughout much of her life. Now, as her memory was failing, she wrote her thoughts out when she felt confused.

At the end of the first week, I offered the sheet to the same Senior who I'd told about the milk.

'It's okay – we don't need that,' she said, with a weak smile, 'we do our care plans after getting to know the person.'

That seems odd, I thought. *I wrote this down to help you get to know Mum and inform your care plans.* I politely persisted and she took the document from me, both of us looking awkward before I walked away. That first taste of dismissal was subtle but clear.

Undeterred, I gave a copy to one of the activity coordinators and stressed how much Mum loved painting and drawing, in the hope that they tried that out first. I looked forward to seeing what happened and, a few days later, popped my head around the door of their office.

'How did the art go?' I smiled, keeping my tone light.

'She can't put pen to paper,' she said, coldly. The words hit me like a slap in the face, but I stepped further into the room.

'What d'you mean?'

'I gave her a piece of paper and a pen, and she couldn't do anything with it.' She stated only the facts, adding no more detail.

I stiffened at her cold response but persisted. 'Oh, that's a shame,' I said, hesitating before I suggested. 'I think she's been very anxious lately – maybe that has affected her. Can we try something else then? Or try another time?'

I wasn't sure exactly what to suggest but I didn't want to leave the conversation at that. Mum loved all things creative, and if anything could soothe her it would be along those lines. *Don't write her off*, I thought, feeling defensive on Mum's behalf. Out of my depth, I decided to leave it for now, but I knew I didn't like what I'd heard. At that point, I knew nothing about adapting activities or creating meaningful experiences. That conversation later spurred me on to embark on a learning path that had a huge impact on my life and ultimately would lead me to change my career. However, back then – I was simply a daughter trying to help her mother. I faked a smile, mumbled a request to keep trying, and left the room.

My focus had to be on helping my nervous mum find her way in this new world. She was uncertain in her surroundings and as such looked for reassurance all the time. She politely asked carers where she was – and why she was there. She worried about having no money to pay for the food when she went for her meals. Busy carers tried to answer her questions and reassure her that everything was paid for, but they always needed to move on to the next resident. Mum, left alone in her room with her jumbled thoughts, was bewildered. Frequently, in those early days, I visited and found her sitting alone without anything to do. She looked lost and lonely again and it broke my heart to see her like that.

Despite the lukewarm response to my previous suggestions, I continued to share what I thought was helpful information. I downloaded the Alzheimer's Society 'This is Me' life history document and hoped that it would have more clout than my basic A4 sheet. Perhaps this would be accepted, read and absorbed by care staff so that they could help Mum become a part of her new home.

That didn't work either, nor did other later attempts. I couldn't know for sure whether carers read those documents but from what I saw, the information I shared wasn't used to establish a routine that suited Mum. Nothing I offered seemed to have any impact on how Mum spent her days.

A few staff appeared indifferent to my efforts. They didn't seem to appreciate that, after years of looking after Mum and coordinating her care packages, it was difficult for me to hand over the reins fully until I was confident that she was okay. I knew that she was safe, well fed and clean, but surely her anxiety needed addressing too. Each tentative attempt to steer carers to think about Mum as an individual was followed by disappointment at their lack of interest in anything I had to say.

My initiation into the care system was a steep learning curve and resulted in uncomfortable insights. It appeared that, by moving to this home, Mum had transformed from an individual into a 'resident' and getting to know her personality and preferences didn't seem a huge priority. They knew what foods she liked but didn't appear as interested in what might soothe her. Of course, I knew that she was only one of lots of residents who needed caring for, but surely this was important. Perhaps this was a symptom of a care system in which staff were too busy to fully apply this vital part of the process. Whatever the reason, it wasn't right, and I couldn't ignore it.

As far as my role went, that seemed no better. I sensed a subtle tone of 'we know best' from staff and I felt disregarded as her daughter. I'm sure they didn't mean to make me feel this way, but I felt like a bystander who needed to know her place and I knew that Aileen felt the same. I suspected that I was overstepping an invisible line that I did not know existed and I would have to learn how to negotiate my way through this 'care home world'.

From staff reactions, I sensed we were gaining a reputation as 'fussy daughters', which felt unfair. It hurt that our genuine efforts seemed to be viewed so cynically and not seen as the natural reactions of worried daughters. Regardless of what I felt, I couldn't focus too long on that. I needed to concentrate on working with the care team to make Mum comfortable and help her to settle into this home.

Chapter 5
'A duck out of water': Bewildered
January 2013

Despite her memory problems, Mum still understood lots of things and her social skills were good. Throughout her life, she'd been timid and shy but visibly bloomed in any situation where she felt accepted. Then, she'd relax, give a coy smile, and use her witty comments to keep everyone entertained. On the other hand, if she felt uneasy, she clammed up and removed herself as soon as she could. We had high hopes that the home was the right environment for her.

In the flat, the front door had become a barrier to Mum mixing with her neighbours and being alone made her more confused and scared. I had imagined that the communal areas with staff and other residents around her most of the time would make her less afraid. I also hoped that her friendly, kind personality meant that she'd quickly bond with others, and she would fit in.

On arriving for each visit, I asked carers how Mum had fared in the previous twenty-four hours since one of us had been there. Any positive response made me feel relieved but a negative one catapulted me into worry that immediately showed on my face. Occasionally, a Senior might report that Mum had been 'unsettled', but they wouldn't seem alarmed. I wanted to know exactly what that meant so probed further and was often confused by the vague responses I got. None the wiser, I assumed that this was part of the normal transition into care home life, but it didn't make me any less worried about my mum.

I looked for the positives and mentally kept a tally. If I heard her joke with one of the carers, I'd add that to the positives list. If carers mentioned that she'd been mixing with other residents I was thrilled and added that too. I was desperate for any evidence of her settling in but also on high alert for signs of things not going so well. I didn't need to look too hard.

There were so many alien aspects to Mum's situation that unnerved her. The home was noisy with the sound of alarms going off every few minutes, which made her jump. The call bells in resident bedrooms, central bathrooms, communal spaces and the front doorbell were all linked to one system, which meant that the alarms went off on every floor simultaneously. I ached as I saw Mum flinch for the umpteenth time at a noise that was unrelated to her floor or merely indicated that someone was at the front door. It created a constant sense of urgency that we both found unsettling.

Mum also struggled with the strangeness of sitting in the communal lounge, watching TV for most of the day with complete strangers. The large neat, but dated, room had chairs placed around the perimeter walls forming a curve and facing towards the TV. No one spoke. People sat close to each other but looked disconnected from each other.

One day, I arrived midmorning to find Mum sitting in the lounge. Her shock of white curly hair hadn't been styled in the usual way and it looked a little frizzy. Her neat purple twinset and woollen skirt peeked out through her open lilac coat that she wore despite being indoors. She saw me approach her chair and greeted me with an indignant look, saying, 'Thank God you're here! I've sat here all day and haven't seen the doctor yet.'

That explains the coat, I thought. *Mam must think she's in a doctor's waiting room.* I wasn't surprised that she felt she'd been waiting around and was frustrated when nothing had happened. In the couple of weeks that she'd lived there I'd noticed that there wasn't much going on in the lounge on a day-to-day basis. It did feel like a waiting room.

'You're not waiting for a doctor, Mam,' I said. 'This is a lounge where everyone who lives here comes and sits together during the day. You know, so you can have some company.'

'Is it?' She looked uncertain.

I looked around for friendly faces and thought of the irony of what I'd said. Everyone kept their head down or stared at the TV. *There's not much company in here,* I thought, perhaps a little unkindly. *Is this how she is going to spend her days?* Disappointment swept over me, but I couldn't let Mum see that. I smiled and offered a 'hello' to a lady who caught my eye, but she turned away without speaking. I looked back towards Mum who looked as if to say, 'see what I mean?' Poor Mum yearned for any smiley face that made her feel at home.

The quiet of the lounge was suddenly interrupted by a lady who started wailing, 'Help me, help me!' She paused for a few seconds and then started again. 'Help me, please help me!' Mum, wide-eyed at the sound of the lady's distress, nudged me with her elbow.

'Do something,' she whispered.

'It's okay, Mam. The carers will help the lady,' I said, feebly, and to my utter relief two carers appeared and took the lady to the bathroom. Within ten minutes of them returning her to the lounge the lady shouted out again. 'Help me, someone please help me!' One of the same carers came to her aid again and tried to soothe her. It worked for a short while before the pleas for help started again. My only option was to keep reassuring Mum that everything was okay. Inside, I did not feel it was okay and she must have sensed this.

'Come on, let's go,' she said. I hesitated for a few minutes until the lady was calm again and then led Mum out of the lounge towards her bedroom. Inside her comfy room, I closed the door and hoped that she'd forget what she'd seen.

That lounge became a swift induction into dementia. My only experience of the illness at close quarters was with Mum and the patients in the hospital over the preceding months. Several people in the lounge seemed the same as Mum but others had more advanced dementia and it unnerved me as much as her. I thought, *If I'm puzzled and scared in this room, God knows what Mam must be feeling.*

Of course, Mum didn't realise why she was in this strange place, surrounded by people with various ailments. She didn't realise that she, herself, had dementia and consequently what she saw and heard seemed odd to her. A few days later, in that same lounge, I sat beside her and she turned to me, summing up her feelings.

'I'm a duck out of water,' she said.

Her words sent shivers through me. Even though she used the wrong word and meant to say 'fish' I thought, *I get it Mam. In your mind, the people in here are different to you and are much more poorly. You don't know what to do here, it's boring and you don't feel comfortable. You don't feel like you belong.* I wanted to help her fit in, but I was still learning about the home myself.

I didn't know what I was supposed to do when I saw or heard someone in distress so opted to check in with staff all the time. 'Excuse me, Mrs X says she needs her mother.' Then later, 'Sorry to bother you but that gentleman said he wants to go home.' The blank looks on carers' faces suggested they were used to these comments, and that they didn't appreciate my unsolicited prompts. Later, I learned all about what these statements might mean and how you could respond to them, but at the time I was a daughter out of her depth and a fellow 'duck out of water.'

Mum feeling awkward was bad enough but there was another lounge-related worry on the horizon. One afternoon, I noticed that one lady – let's call her 'Mrs B' – sat near the door and shouted at other residents, telling them to sit down whenever they got up from their chairs. This went on repeatedly, with frightened residents complying and staff interjecting but to no real effect. Mum's eyes darted between Mrs B and others as if she was watching a horror show – it made my stomach churn. *Thank God Mam hasn't caught her attention,* I thought and was immediately ashamed of thinking that way. I was stuck in a no-win situation: watch someone get shouted at and do nothing or keep raising it with the carers and get on their nerves. I chose the latter. Again, I reassured Mum that it was fine, and she wasn't in any danger. It wasn't fine and I hadn't a clue what to do to make it better longer term.

*****

Against such an unsettling backdrop, of course Mum wanted to go home and, after each visit, she asked if I could take her with me when I left. 'Our Helen – how about I come home now?' or 'Will you take me to your house with you?' She asked in such a gentle way that it tore at my heart to refuse her.

'Sorry Mam, the doctor said you need to stay here for a while.'

I kept thinking about her little flat where she had been contented for the last eight years and how she would be devastated if she knew it wasn't there any more. The deceit burned into my stomach even though I knew I couldn't do as she asked. I only rationalised it by reminding myself that even when she was living in her own flat, dementia meant that she frequently yearned for an elusive place that gave her the feeling of home.

*****

The worries continued. Another resident, Mrs H, who in the first few days greeted Mum with a friendly smile, had changed her feelings. She no longer saw Mum as a friend, and frequently let her know about a perceived wrongdoing. Eventually, even seeing Mrs H in the corridor scared Mum and if she had to walk past her, she steered her walking frame as far away from her as she could. Sometimes that worked but sometimes the verbal assault took place anyway. I hoped dementia meant that Mum soon forgot. She didn't.

One day, as we sat together in her bedroom, Mum saw Mrs H pass by the door. I prayed she would move on without stopping but shouted a cheery 'hello' anyway. Mum pulled me close to her and said, 'she doesn't like me'.

I tried to reassure her – 'Oh, I think she might be a bit poorly, Mum,' – but this didn't allay her fears. Mum didn't understand the reason for the ill-will between them, was frightened of her and hadn't forgotten any of the incidents.

I knew I had to do something about this but, of course, I was aware that Mrs H was also living with dementia so wasn't purposefully being aggressive. The good news was that this lady had a lovely daughter and we'd had a few friendly chats in the first couple of weeks. We were both mortified at the unpleasantness we'd witnessed between our mums, but knew the limitations that dementia brought. One afternoon, I saw the daughter in the communal kitchen and suggested that all four of us could have a cuppa together one day. I thought if our respective parents saw that everyone was friendly then there was nothing to worry about. It seemed like a good idea.

Meanwhile, I mentioned my concerns to the carers and asked them to keep an eye on things between Mum and Mrs H. I later regretted having had both of those conversations.

Chapter 6
'Back off': The Warning
January 2013

Twenty-four days after Mum moved into the care home, the manager rang me for what I, at first, assumed was a general chat. *How nice, I thought.*

After discussing a few general points, she went on to tell me that I needed to 'back off from staff and let them do their job'. A flash of embarrassment ran through me as I realised the reason for the call.

I was mortified at the thought of causing any upset and explained to the manager that hadn't been my intention. I wracked my brain for what I could have said or done wrong, and asked her for an example so that I didn't make the same mistake again. Apparently, I'd been asking carers lots of questions, wanted to see care records and, worse still, had a conversation with another relative which had caused offence. It seemed that my general curiosity – a long-standing trait – was putting staff under pressure and having an effect on morale.

This list of unintentional misdemeanours seemed a little harsh, but I knew that this wasn't a good start to our time at the home. I repeated my apology and asked for it to be relayed back to carers – I wanted to make amends.

Before ending the call, she made sure that I understood the consequences of me not complying by explaining that, if things didn't change, she would have to ask Mum to leave. My heart hit the floor. *What have I done?* We had already handed in the keys from Mum's council flat so she couldn't go back there. The prospect of her being uprooted from this new place to God-knows-where horrified me. I fumed at myself for having put her safety in jeopardy by being my usual curious self and asking too many questions.

I was embarrassed and terrified but knew I had to tell my sisters of the warning and, more importantly, make sure that Aileen didn't find herself in the same boat. I immediately called her. In a sisterly show of support, Aileen tried to comfort me. She was more objective and helped me reflect on the events of the previous three weeks and why I had acted in a particular way. The driving factor for everything either of us had said or done was trying to help our anxious Mum settle in.

But alone, I ruminated even more about which questions were the problem. *Was it the questions about how the home worked? Was it when I asked about how she was spending her day? Was it when I asked about Mam's nervousness and what they were doing about it? Surely these are reasonable – aren't they?* I examined everything but could only come to a troubling conclusion about how the home had handled this situation.

We were all inexperienced with these new living arrangements, and surely it was natural for any relative to turn to carers for information and reassurance. I thought about the care team's own part in this miscommunication. If they had provided me with the relevant information in the first place, I wouldn't have needed to ask all those questions. Aileen and I had spent three weeks simply seeking their advice and trying to orientate our mother and ourselves into a new and confusing world.

I now felt annoyed at the manager's defensive position. She knew that Mum, the home's newest resident, was having difficulties and that it was natural for us to worry about her. My thoughts turned to her leadership: *Where is her empathy? What is she doing to help staff to support Mam, and us? Would she usually threaten someone within less than a month?*

Regardless of what I thought, the phone call had its desired effect in reducing the number of questions I asked in the coming days. However, it also increased how uncomfortable I felt. Mum was still nervous and confused but, because of that early threat, I tiptoed around issues and was now afraid to ask any questions. I had no clue what, in their eyes, was a wrong question or deemed to be overstepping the line. I knew Aileen felt the same. I developed an apologetic, deferential stance that I've since seen lots of families adopt. My requests, which had always been polite, now had a hesitancy to them: 'If you've got a minute could you ...?', 'Would it be alright if I ...?'

I hated how this made me feel and knew it wasn't right.

I couldn't continue this way. I felt hard done by and so I asked for a meeting with the manager – on the pretext of having a general review, but I knew I would raise the bigger issue of how the warning had made me feel.

On the day of the meeting, Aileen was working so I asked Ian to attend with me for moral support. This cautious approach was not my style at all, but I was so nervous about the outcome I needed him around. In my professional life, I had navigated many a difficult meeting, but this felt different and the warning had shaken my confidence.

The meeting started with pleasantries, and we covered general points about Mum's care. Eventually, I broached the issue of how I had felt since the phone call and how it had made me behave. I braced myself for a difficult conversation but, to my surprise, the manager apologised for making me feel that way. She reassured me that I could ask any question necessary, and she would do her best to make sure things improved. *That was easier than I imagined,* I thought. *Okay – let's move forward.* We agreed to meet regularly to keep things on track and I was grateful that the manager had understood. But, as we said our goodbyes, I couldn't shift a niggling worry about how things seemed to work in the home.

*****

My steep learning curve around care home life continued and, ironically, it was my poorly mother who helped me see things more clearly. One day when I visited her, she was agitated.

'I don't like this job,' she said. 'I don't know what to do.'

She was, of course, referring to her feelings of being confused in the care home. She felt weirdly out of place, she didn't know what was expected of her and felt she didn't fit in.

While she spoke in the wrong context, her words reminded me that she (and we) had been plunged unexpectedly into this new world which had similarities to when someone starts a new job. As I compared the two scenarios, it helped me make sense of our rocky start.

In a new job, you have a period of induction. This helps you get to know 'how things are done around here'. You are introduced to your co-workers and, in a good organisation, supported to develop positive relationships. You have an opportunity to learn about the people and their roles, you get to know about the routines, when things happen and what is expected of you.

Entering care home life is similar in that it means that there is a whole new way of doing things for residents and their families. It struck me that neither Mum nor my sister or I were offered much in the way of an introduction to this unfamiliar world and so we had done all we could to find our own way. We were learning. We were building relationships and having to do it on our own. We needed to be supported, not admonished.

Mum needed help to get to know her fellow residents. The relationship between her and the care staff needed to be developed with respect and dignity. Only if these were in place would Mum start to feel like she belonged there. The relationship between us as a family, the manager and care staff needed clear two-way communication for us to feel we were 'in this together'. It couldn't include a limit on the number of questions we asked or censorship on our part. For this to work as a long-term relationship, our interactions had to be natural and free flowing.

I needed to be part of Mum's new life in the care home. I needed to have an easy relationship with those who were caring for her and have an equal position to them in our joint caring role. I didn't want to feel like a visitor who came in with gifts and no more than a 'how's Mum?' by way of conversation. I wanted to feel that I was truly part of her care and I resolved that this was the way it had to be.

Alongside this, I realised there were unspoken rules on how I was allowed to be involved in her care. The consequences of me not playing by their rules had been spelt out clearly. In any other situation, I was bold enough to make my point and stand up for what was right. I now knew that in 'care home world' I had to tread carefully as I did this. It wasn't me who was ultimately disadvantaged if I didn't toe the line – it was Mum. The risk was real; I now knew the score and I felt afraid.

This fear stayed with me, one way or another, for the next seven years.

Chapter 7
'Please help me!': The Phone Calls
February 2013

Mum loved chatting to people. In person was best but, if that wasn't possible, she loved chatting on the phone. At home in the '80s and '90s, Dad used to moan to her about the cost of her lengthy calls. She viewed the evidence on the phone bills, made apologetic noises but then carried on having long chats with her friends.

Years later, phone calls from my sister, Barbara, in Australia were a regular feature for Mum. They talked happily for hours about everything and, despite the miles between them, they stayed closely connected to each other's lives. Dementia eventually curtailed the length of calls as Mum couldn't sustain the conversation, but they were still important to her.

The phone became her lifeline in other ways. Initially, Mum needed a bit of reassurance when she got muddled, but as her memory got worse, the calls became more urgent and spanned all hours of the day and night. Despite them giving me sleepless nights, I was comforted in knowing that, if she was afraid, she always let us know.

So, of course, when Mum moved to the care home, we immediately had a telephone installed in her bedroom allowing her to stay in touch with all three daughters. This turned out to be both a blessing and a curse. If those calls from the flat had provided an occasional window into her thoughts, the months ahead became a real eye-opener. Mum called us daily from the care home. Numerous times.

The calls varied in their message, tone and intensity. At best, there were occasional 'keep-in-touch' calls where Mum's mood seemed light. 'What's happening today, our Helen?' she'd say, and be happy with an explanation.

Increasingly, though, there were the confused calls asking, 'Where am I?', or a frustrated 'I'm sick of this place!' At times there was an escalation from one level to another in a matter of hours. The most troubling were the frightened calls when Mum was overcome with panic and begged, 'Please, help me!'

Whatever the call, I kept my voice bright and breezy and my responses light and reassuring. I believed that if, she heard me sounding relaxed, she'd feel that everything was okay. She couldn't know that I felt very differently.

The phone calls usually started around 9.30 am and, depending on their content, set my mood for the day. I lived on a knife-edge and my days were ruled by the unpredictability of dementia and how it affected Mum. I tried to establish a routine but never knew how she would feel and, consequently, where I would end up. I couldn't focus on my work properly so didn't pursue any new projects. I didn't have the headspace – I felt I had to concentrate on helping Mum settle into this home.

One morning, I had planned on doing some admin at home and had arranged to visit Mum the following day. The phone rang. I knew it was her and felt the familiar knot in my stomach. *Please God, let her be okay today.* I lifted the receiver towards my ear, but could hear she was already talking.

'Our Helen – I'm lost,' she said, alarm rising in her voice.

'No Mam – don't worry – you're in the right place.' I tried to slow her fear down. 'I'll explain everything.' I launched into the routine that we, her daughters, had agreed between us. 'You are in a new flat, Mam. Remember, you broke your knee?

'Did I?' she said, sounding unconvinced.

'Yes, and the doctors said that they wanted you to live somewhere that has carers around to help you. The room you are in now is your 'bedsit flat' and that is where you live now.'

'Oh, I see.' Her tone was so trusting – I winced at my half-deception.

We had been advised to keep the explanation for her moving house as near to the truth as possible without specifically mentioning her dementia. Yes, the doctors and social workers did want her to have 24-hour care, but it was because of both her physical *and* her memory problems. We wanted her to still feel independent, so agreed that we would call the care home a 'block of flats' and her bedroom the 'bedsit' or 'flat.'

'The good thing is, Mam, you are *never* on your own there.' I hoped that this extra bit of information helped her feel safe. 'But either me or Aileen comes to see you every day and Barbara can phone you whenever she likes.'

'Are you sure?'

'Yes, Mam, is that okay?'

This seemed to satisfy her, and she agreed to stay there. We said our goodbyes and hung up. I knew it didn't feel like home yet but hoped that she would settle in soon.

Of course, my reassurances didn't last long as she forgot what I had said and called back a few minutes later. I reassured her again and she accepted my explanation once more. Within thirty minutes the phone rang for the third time. I closed my eyes as my stomach lurched again – hearing her voice more insistent this time.

'Our Helen – you need to come and get me. I'm lost. Please!'

'No, Mam – don't worry – you're in the right place.'

'I'm not! Please – come and get me – now!' she begged.

I was about to launch into those well-rehearsed lines again but stopped myself. *What are you doing? She's scared and this isn't working – you need to go to see her.* Not for the first time, I wrestled with the need to get on with my day and the urge to go to her side. This was a chaotic and unpredictable way to live but I knew what came next.

'Don't worry, Mam, I'm on my way.'

My need to make things right for her was too strong. I grabbed my bag, jumped in the car and raced towards the home, arriving fifteen minutes later.

As the lift doors opened, I bumped into one of the carers, who looked surprised to see me. 'I thought you were coming tomorrow?' she said.

'I know, but I've had three panicky calls this morning – that's why I've come up. Is she okay?'

'She was fine last time I went in,' she said. 'She was laughing and joking when I took her a cup of tea.'

'Let's see how she is now,' I said, and hurried towards Mum's room.

From the doorway of her bedroom, I could see her perched on the edge of the chair, looking ready to bolt. Worry knotted her eyebrows, as she gazed at the floor, pondering what to do next. She looked up, saw me and let out a sigh. 'Thank God you're here,' she said.

'It's okay, Mam. You're okay.' As I walked towards her, I noticed that the basket of her walking frame was stuffed with her clothes. *She's been packing again,* I thought.

I reached over, planting a kiss on her cheek.

'I've got myself muddled,' she said.

'Don't worry, Mam. Let's get you comfortable on here first.' I eased her back onto the chair. 'We can sort this out.'

I held her hand for a little while, repeating the explanations for why she lived there, and answering her questions.

Once she was calmer, I changed the focus by finding us something practical to do. Just like we had when she lived in the flat, we unpacked the contents of the basket so they could be returned to the drawers she had emptied a few hours before. She meticulously rolled or folded each item of underwear, passing them to me when she felt they were ready to be returned to their rightful place. Her shoulders dropped as she relaxed, and a faint smile returned to her lips as we chatted. *Panic over.*

After a while, she closed her eyes and dozed off. I took the opportunity to head to the communal kitchen and explain the morning's events to the carer who, in turn, shared her version. I knew that both of our accounts, although conflicting, were true. I had seen Mum before, frightened or weepy one minute and then saying a cheery 'hello' to a carer the next. She often hid her worries from them, and the sudden changes in her mood were confusing for all of us.

Back in her room, I watched Mum sleep, studying the now peaceful face that despite her eighty-plus years still had few wrinkles. *I wish you had a friend here, Mam,* I thought, s*omeone to sit with you so you don't feel alone.* Of course, carers popped into her room now and then, chatting briefly, but they were busy and needed to move on. Left alone for long periods with nothing to do, she became confused. She must have wondered where on earth she was – and the calls to us were her only way of getting reassurance. The phone was still her lifeline.

*****

Mum knew Aileen's phone number off by heart so, when she panicked, she automatically called her first. Aileen was at usually at work so the call went to voicemail, and she'd leave a message. Having got no response there she would then try my number and I took over. Poor Aileen would come home for her lunchtime break to several distressed messages that, of course, made her anxious and affected her day. We spoke about it but couldn't resolve the dilemma: Mum needed a phone in her room so that Barbara could have contact with her, but the countless calls were adding to Aileen's stress. I felt sorry for my sister, but I was stuck and didn't know what to do.

As the months rolled on, the distraught calls and voicemails continued multiple times a day. The phone dilemma and other worries about Mum's care led to arguments between Aileen and me and our relationship was tense. We bickered about what was the best course of action and seldom agreed. In a resentful moment, I analysed Mum's phone bills which showed how many calls each of us were getting. It was a petty and pointless thing to do, but it did illustrate, through the sheer volume of calls, how often Mum was anxious. This helped me make the case to the manager that Mum was still not settling in, but I also needed to stop the calls to Aileen. *I must fix this.*

I found a solution when I came across a solid Perspex picture frame in a local store. I wrote my phone numbers in large print with the message: 'Rita – if worried, ring Helen.' I placed the frame on the windowsill right next to the phone thinking that Mum would see this first and call me instead of Aileen. It worked, and Aileen started to receive less calls, but the obvious result was that now I got more. Hearing her distress multiple times a day, regardless of whether I was at the care home or at my house, heightened my own anxiety.

I was permanently on high alert and the mere sound of my phone ringing caused me to tense up. I wanted to help Mum, but knew that dashing up to the care home every time she reached out wasn't the right solution and it couldn't go on. In a conversation with a kindly dementia support advisor, they suggested that Mum needed to learn to rely on the carers more for her day-to-day reassurances. I knew they were right but wasn't sure how I could get this to happen. Ironically, there was a bright orange call button in her room that, if pressed, sounded the alarm alerting carers that she needed assistance. Of course, dementia meant that she didn't remember it was there and, even if she had, she wouldn't know how to use it.

I needed another solution and tried to untangle the problem with logic: Mum didn't feel at home yet and if she thought she was in this mysterious building alone she became scared. However, if she saw the carers around her, she was reassured that she was safe and that feeling seemed to last for a while. If I could build on the feeling of safety and reduce the amounts of time between bouts of panic, then she might start to relax. It was a shame that, whenever she panicked, she reached for the phone and not the call button. *That's it!* I thought, *she doesn't know how to use the call button but does know how to use a phone.*

With the manager's permission, I placed the call button on the windowsill right next to the phone and the Perspex frame. My thinking went like this: when Mum felt scared, she would ring me. I would talk her through how to press the orange button and wait until a carer came to respond. I would then ask Mum to hand the phone to them, explain her worries, and they could reassure her. *Brilliant!* I thought, *it's just a different way to use the call button.*

Sometimes, the plan worked perfectly, and, between us, we managed to soothe my distressed mother. Other days, I bellowed down the phone, 'Mam! Press the orange button!' only for her to say, 'I can't see it.'

'Next to the phone, Mam. Look down!'

Carers must have thought I was mad, but I was happy that we had a solution that worked, even partially. Those who went along with this make-do system saved my sanity, and we celebrated our successes. Others appeared cold to the idea and seemed to miss that I was trying to ease Mum's distress as it happened. Whenever I got puzzled looks, I kept saying, 'it's just a different way to help Mam use the call button.' I was frustrated by their indifference or, worse still, when I felt I was not supported at all.

On a few visits, the Perspex frame was missing or in various places around the room. I felt uneasy about this but couldn't be sure that Mum hadn't moved it, so I kept returning it to its place. One day I found it in tucked away in a drawer and asked the Senior on duty if they could make sure the frame was kept within Mum's eyesight.

'D'you think it might be seeing your phone number that upsets your mam?' she suggested.

'Mmm – I don't think so,' I said. 'From what I've noticed, Mam is upset first, then tries to get in touch with us – I don't think it is seeing the number that does it.'

My stiff smile probably didn't hide my annoyance at her immediately defaulting to a negative stance. She didn't respond so I filled the silence.

'I know everyone is so busy here and carers might not always see that she is scared.' I didn't want it to sound as if I was blaming anyone. 'This is just a way that she can let you know that she needs help,' I said, trying to keep the focus on helping Mum.

The Senior made vague comments about Mum's distress being part of the settling-in process but, even at this early stage, I knew that we could do more to keep her calm and happy. Despite my earlier warning from the manager, I tentatively suggested that Mum needed company and stimulation so that she wasn't afraid. She was spending a lot of time alone in her room and that seemed to lead to worried thinking.

'We don't offer one-to-one care,' she said.

I'd heard this type of stock response before, when I'd asked about something else, and once again it stung.

'No – of course not. Just … if we can help her to mix more.'

'We'll try,' she said. With a few more platitudes she went on her way, leaving me brooding.

She doesn't bloody need one-to-one care, I thought. *She needs help to feel less anxious here. Can't you see that?*

Once again, I felt misunderstood, and this wasn't my only grumble.

Earlier niggles around some aspects of care had started to grow. The carers were very experienced and treated Mum nicely, but they were also fixed in their ways. They did things the way they had always done them – and some things didn't work for Mum. Too often, I needed to point out things that had been missed: support stockings, waist slips and other items left off made her feel half-dressed and uncomfortable. Giving her water to wash down her pills (rather than the milk we had agreed on several times) made her blanch at the bitter taste. Omissions around the bathroom routine had more considerable effects and minor issues could escalate quickly into Mum having a difficult day. To someone living with dementia, it is important to keep to an agreed familiar routine and I couldn't ignore the inconsistencies I observed.

I had nagging doubts about communication in the home. Messages weren't passed on and I had to repeat requests several times to various Seniors. It was awkward but I tried to keep my tone relaxed – inside I felt growing frustration.

I was saddened to think that living in a care home was bringing Mum little solace. I clung on to the knowledge that, despite the tough time she was having, the anxious episodes did pass, and she would be momentarily happy again. This might be within the next hour, day or week. Whenever she felt better, I did too.

Besides, we were dealing with so many other health issues that my head spun.

Chapter 8

'I must pull myself together': The Creaking Gate

March 2013

Our 'creaking gate' was doing a lot more than creaking by now, as Mum's physical health worsened alongside the memory problems. The fixer in me was determined to help her, but I struggled to know what to tackle first. There was so much to keep track of that I kept an ongoing list that I checked regularly with whichever Senior was on duty.

Top of my list was anything toilet-related, which dominated the early months in the care home. As Mum switched between periods of constipation, diarrhoea and UTIs, she was permanently uncomfortable which made her even more anxious. She fretted about keeping herself clean, changing her underwear and replacing pads. She couldn't remember where these were kept in her bedroom, so I asked for spares to be left in the bathroom. As before, I encouraged her to drink lots of water to prevent further UTIs but, of course, that meant more frequent trips to the toilet. At first, she was able to go independently but, as panic and dementia took over, she couldn't manage this basic personal task alone. My self-conscious mum allowed me or Aileen to help her with toilet matters but, at that stage, refused help from the carers and muddled through unaided – with mixed results.

A carer approached me one day, blocking my way as I got out of the lift. 'Your mam has been stuffing toilet paper into her knickers,' she said, with a hint of accusation in her tone.

'Has she?

'Yes – she's been putting extra knickers on as well,' she continued, as if adding more wrongdoings. Rattled at her tell-tale voice, I adopted my 'Rita defence' mode.

'Well – if she doesn't think she's got any pads handy, she's probably trying to protect them from getting wet,' I said. 'She would be mortified if she had an 'accident.'

'Yeah – probably ...' She hesitated as I edged past her to get to Mum's room.

Sounds perfectly logical to me, I thought, *how come YOU haven't thought of that?*

Sadly, I often found Mum mortified at having had another 'accident' and it broke my heart to see her so humiliated.

On another day, soon after I'd arrived, I noticed Mum wriggling in her chair and stamping her feet a few times on the floor. These were tell-tale signs that she either needed to go to the toilet soon or that it was too late, and she needed help changing. That day it was the latter.

'Let's nip to the loo, Mam,' I said, prompting her to heave herself from her chair and make our way into the compact bathroom. This had become a familiar routine: Mum sat on the loo, with me crouched down beside her, nattering away as I did the necessary freshen up. She bit the side of her lip as she looked down at me.

'I'm sorry, pet,' she said. 'You shouldn't have to do this.' Her shame filled the tiny space.

'No problem, Mam,' I told her brightly. 'We're all girls together. I can have this done in a jiffy!'

'I know, but you shouldn't have to,' she said.

'That's okay, Mam – it only takes two minutes. Before you know it, we'll be back in your room, nice and comfortable with a cup of tea.'

After the deed was done, I manoeuvred Mum and her walking frame around the tight squeeze in the bathroom to wash our hands and make our way back into the bedroom. She hesitated, putting her hand on my arm. 'I don't know what I'd do without you.' I felt my heart lurch. She often said this, and I responded with my now-usual reply.

'You don't have to, Mam; I'll always be here!' I pecked her on the cheek and grinned as she plonked down heavily into the chair. Once she was clean and dry we could relax with the memory of the accident and (hopefully) any embarrassment fading.

Further down the dementia line, Mum couldn't tell me what was making her uncomfortable. She could tell me that something wasn't right, but her brain simply couldn't locate the source. In these instances, I used a process of elimination to detect the problem and the first thing I did was to rule out any toilet issue. Whenever that was resolved we had a chance of her being settled.

As a result, I became hypervigilant about toilet issues. I reasoned that if being physically uncomfortable was adding to her difficulties, then between us (me, Aileen and the carers) we should at least be able to get that right. This began a long mission to keep Mum clean and dry that turned into a minefield.

Apparently, moving from independent living to care home and from one local authority area to another ultimately meant fewer and less absorbent pads. I felt aggrieved but resorted to buying our own supply of 'posh pads' for outdoor trips. More complex challenges came along later, but for now the 'posh pads' solved an immediate problem and I asked the carers to prompt Mum regularly about going to the loo.

*****

Next on my list was Mum's diabetes. Thankfully, most aspects were well-managed with daily visits from the district nurse for insulin injections. However, her long-standing troubles with her feet and poor circulation had flared up and, as a diabetic, this was a concern. Previously she had six-weekly appointments with the local NHS podiatry team which had kept bigger problems at bay.

However, as with the pad situation, her change in living circumstances disrupted that well-established foot care routine. I was informed that she needed a brand-new referral and that arrangements for people in care homes differed significantly. I grappled with the system and made repeated phone calls to get treatment for her sore toes, puffy feet and swollen legs. I was mystified by the bureaucracy that meant unnecessary delays in her continued care. In years to come the new arrangements worked like a dream and were an example of great care, but getting us into the system took a while.

*****

Other sporadic health issues appeared, and I added them to the ever-growing list. Every few weeks, Mum complained of chest pains and asked to see a doctor. As she had a history of angina, this needed to be taken seriously and always meant a trip to the Accident & Emergency department of the local hospital. I would drop whatever I was doing to join Mum there and thankfully each time the pain would eventually subside. After hours of waiting, while busy medical teams concentrated on more needy patients, eventually it would be Mum's turn for an X-Ray. The results were the same each time – they couldn't see anything wrong with Mum's heart and assumed it must be a muscular issue. Although this was good news, we would return to the care home, both feeling frazzled after our lengthy wait. After several trips with the same result, Aileen and I asked Mum's GP to make a note on her records to stop taking her to hospital with chest pains, as we knew there was no serious medical cause. We prayed that this wasn't a mistake on our part.

When someone goes into a care home, the care team take the responsibility for ninety per cent of the communication with their GP. I was happy to hand over the responsibility but felt one step behind the care staff in understanding what was going on. I tried to keep track with my endless lists, but my frequent questions, their vague responses and the sheer volume of issues made my head spin.

When friends enquired about Mum, my response was flippant. 'If it's not her bum it's her feet. If it's not her feet, it's her heart. If it's not her heart, it's her head. I literally don't know if I'm dealing with her arse or her elbow!'

I also joked that I was going to write a book about how I was keeping track of everything about my mother. My list went from the top of her head right down to her toes and everything in between. 'It's not going to be called *From Here to Eternity*, I said. 'It'll be *From Pads to Podiatry*'. The name stuck and in fact I use that title for a chapter later in this book.

Despite my outward humour, the reality was no joke. Mum had endured countless health challenges in her life and *now* her rapidly declining memory was stealing her thoughts – and she knew it.

At first, whenever she forgot a word or lost the thread of a conversation, she'd ask, 'why can't I remember things?' I'd often say, 'don't worry, Mam, leave it for now and it'll come back to you'. Even after her diagnosis, we never used the word dementia as we knew it would frighten her. Instead, we talked of her being 'forgetful' but, as problems occurred more often, she'd wail, 'what's wrong with me?' My reassurances only helped in the short term and, as her thoughts became increasingly jumbled, she even questioned her own sanity: 'Am I going daft?'

She tried so hard to make sense of a world that had become so frightening for her – even trying to explain the panic she felt – 'I get a fizzy feeling and then something goes wrong.'

One morning, she announced, 'I must pull myself together.' I'd heard these words when I was younger, whenever she was feeling depressed. She had always willed herself to power through her unhappiness to do whatever needed to be done. She overcame so many hurdles, but it was only once I was an adult that I realised how strong she must have been. Now, in the care home, she tried to apply that same determination, promising that she would try her hardest to get better. *Oh, Mam,* I thought, *this is something you can't fix. It's now down to us to help you stay well.*

She was tortured and it was agony to watch. *This is so unfair – she has put up with so much in her life already – and now this.* I agonised over the list of ailments and how I could manage things better, but I knew I was firefighting.

Chapter 9

'The Lord is My Shepherd': Back to Church

April 2013

Mum needed to adapt to this new life, but, at the same time, needed the comfort of some familiar routines. Her Christian faith, and regularly attending church, had soothed her through life's difficulties – I wondered if it could help her now. Going back to church on a Sunday would at least get her out of the care home for a couple of hours.

When Mum (Church of England) married Dad (a Roman Catholic) she had promised to raise her children in his faith. As kids, we had gone to church at Dad's insistence but as teenagers had stopped and were in no hurry to return. Thankfully, a few of Mum's old church friends agreed to help by looking after her during the service. Aileen and I took turns each week driving her there, settling her into her seat and then returning an hour later to take her back to the care home.

The arrangement worked well, and we were grateful for friends' help, but after a while I noticed that Mum became increasingly nervous whenever I attempted to leave. One day, she pleaded with me to stay, and I promised I would. My church days resumed, as quickly as that.

The Sunday routine was carefully orchestrated and needed a team effort for it to work well. We had to arrive at church by 9.50 am if we were to use the entrance next to the car park – any later, and that door was closed. This would mean a long walk around the whole building to the front door which, with Mum's poor mobility, was too difficult.

I confirmed with carers that we needed to leave no later than 9.30 am, so asked if they could have her ready by 9.00 am when I would arrive. Ready, to us, meant smart clothes and her hair neatly combed. Aileen usually styled Mum's hair the day before, so it only needed touching up by the carers.

Aileen had been a hairdresser prior to her current job and had taken pride in doing Mum's hair for as long as I could remember. Although her hair was fine and wispy, she had lots of it and her shock of neat white curls became her trademark.

My job was to carry out the last-minute task of packing her handbag with the necessary 'going out kit'. By now, we had various kits depending on our different excursions. For church, it contained lipstick, tissues, a purse with coins for the collection plate, and the ever-present continence paraphernalia. Oh, and a bag of Quavers for the return journey.

On the Sundays when the routine worked well, I was delighted. On others, when I arrived to find that we were running behind, there was race against the clock, with all hands on deck to get her ready. On those days, I found myself scrambling around the room, grabbing items and stuffing them into the bag. In my head, I could hear the speeded-up music from the 1970s Benny Hill comedy sketches and, with more than a bit of luck, we were generally out the door on time and ready to go to church. Over time we got more organised and, a year or so later, wonderful carers made the routine work like clockwork.

*****

The day that I first agreed to stay at church with Mum, I dreaded the tedious hour that I assumed lay ahead. *What have I got myself into now?* I thought. *I gave this up ages ago.*

Yet, during those sixty minutes, I watched her transform from the person she had become in the care home. There, she was full of doubt and worry, but here in the church she was confident. She knew the order of service off by heart and recited each prayer, word-perfect, without referring to the service sheets. Each time the vicar spoke, she responded – at precisely the right time – keeping up with the rest of the congregation.

Hymns proved a bit more difficult as they were new trendier versions unfamiliar to Mum and, of course, different from those I remembered from the Catholic church. I scrambled for the right place in the hymn book and guided her by pointing to each word. We grinned at each other, as we lurched through each verse not knowing the tune or the key, and I'm sure we sounded terrible. It didn't matter. We sang our hearts out together.

In that familiar environment, she understood where she was and what she was supposed to do. The church service was fixed in her core being and the worries of memory loss seemed to fade away. Her whole body relaxed and, as it did, her playful side re-emerged. Mum's poor mobility meant that she sat down for the whole service, positioned in between me and one of her friends. When I stood up, she tickled the back of my legs. Later she pinched the arm of the friend on the other side. Further into the service, she pulled funny faces at others as they caught her eye to try to make them laugh. I grinned at seeing the mischievous side she still had in her.

The experience was a joy and a revelation. *She can be happy!* I thought. We had spent months watching her struggle emotionally, with only fleeting moments of happiness. Seeing the positive effect on her was encouraging and worth the tiny bit of effort it took for me to accompany her. She found a place that was comforting and, it seemed, so did I.

Over time, I started to enjoy the experience myself and tried my best to listen to the message in the sermon. I was less interested in the formal stuff and found myself tuning out and having my own chat with God.

What's going to happen to Mam? What can I do?

And then pleading.

Please God, help her? Let her get settled in this home.

Regardless of my beliefs, I was ready to plead with any higher power.

Straight after the service, parishioners met in the adjoining church hall for refreshments, and I hoped that chatting with her old pals would do Mum good. As we walked into the hall, people flocked around her, asking how she was keeping and wishing her well. She beamed as she recognised a familiar face, or someone hugged her. I saw how Rita, who had been an important part of this community for decades, was still much loved here.

I met a lady who told me that she and Mum were in the same class at school seventy years earlier. As they sat close to each other with their hands firmly clasped together a wave of pride washed over me. *She has so much history with these people. They know her and care about her – she can feel it!* While they enjoyed a cup of tea, I resolved that I would keep bringing her back here to find that familiar comfort. It was the least that I could do.

Of course, it wasn't all plain sailing. Difficulties arose when well-meaning friends asked questions that challenged Mum's failing memory. Her polite social skills initially masked the decline but anything that went beyond a here-and-now question, such as 'How are you?', left her stumped.

Innocent questions such as, 'Do you like the home?' or 'What's your new place like?' confused her and she'd look to me for the answer. I tried to rescue the situation but struggled to find words that tactfully explained that Mum simply couldn't remember those things any more, and in a way that didn't make her feel foolish. Treading that line, in this and other situations, was a constant challenge for me and I don't know if I ever got it right. Saying nothing, using knowing smiles or 'fudging' the answers was my only way around it. On a good day, I found the right sentence that moved the conversation on. On a bad day, I resorted to whispers and gestures out of Mum's earshot which felt disloyal, regardless of my good intentions. Most of the time these were harmless blips and I hoped that she'd forget the stumbles and move on. That wasn't always the case.

One Sunday, Mum was chatting to a close friend after the service.

'How's Fred?' Mum said.

'Fred?' The friend stared in disbelief. 'He's been dead for years!'

'Is he? Mum said. 'Eeh, I'm really sorry – I didn't know.'

'Of course you did, Rita. He's been dead for donkey's years!' Surprisingly, the friend didn't seem upset at the error and they chatted a bit longer before she moved on.

Mum glanced sideways at me, bit her lip and shook her head.

'How did I not know that?' she asked, incredulously.

'Don't worry, Mam, we all get things wrong,' I said.

As we moved through the hall, she continued to shake her head, as if to say 'What have I done this time?'

That bad feeling a person gets when they have 'put their foot in it' was intensified a hundred times for Mum by the sense of having got it wrong yet again. She, like many people with dementia, was aware of her mistakes. Even when she couldn't remember the details later – it created an uncomfortable feeling that lingered.

That day, my reassurances felt lame. As we drove back to the care home, I could tell from her subdued demeanour that the uneasy feeling remained with her.

*****

The benefits of our church visits were clear to me but there were practical hurdles to overcome. The escalating toilet troubles made preventing any 'accidents' a priority but the church's options were limited.

If we tried the accessible toilet, near to the front door of the church hall, Mum would exclaim, 'I can't 'go' in here – people can hear me!' However, if we used the communal toilets, located further away, she worried about getting locked in the building. Once, halfway through proceedings, she panicked and scrambled to pull her underwear up, ready to dash out of the cubicle. 'We've got to go!' she said, fear gripping her voice. I tried to reassure her, but she was so certain of the impending danger that I had no choice but to swiftly comply with her instruction. I took a deep breath and hoped that 'spending a penny' could wait until we got home.

For me, every outing was split between watching Mum's every move, anticipating what might happen next and swiftly reacting to whatever curveball came our way. From the moment we arrived, until the moment we left, I was second-guessing our next manoeuvre and how to negotiate it: *How can I get her across this bumpy car park? Which loo today? Where are we sitting?* I needed the arms of an octopus to juggle walking frames, doors and handbags, plus a wobbly mother.

Once inside, I tried to anticipate any potential pitfalls in conversation, confusion around the collection plate (when she looked at it blankly) and how to help her with Holy Communion. I was always one or two steps ahead – it was exhausting.

Despite all this, going to church showed me what was still possible for Mum. She could be confident, she could still do lots of practical things, she could relax. I'd seen her contented when I'd taken her to a café, but that was when there were only the two of us. This was more proof that there *were* other situations in which Mum could thrive and be happy. It gave me hope for her future and I knew I had to build on that.

*****

The church routine went on successfully for a few years but, eventually, it became stressful for Mum to attend. As her dementia progressed, she struggled more with words and lost her way. She refused to get out of the car, saying 'I don't like it here,' but couldn't tell me why. Once, in a moment of clarity, she said, 'I feel stupid – I don't know what to say.'

'Don't worry, Mam, I'll help.' Despite my offer, the bad feelings associated with church had started and they didn't go away. It was time to rethink.

At the same time, Mum started to enjoy a lie-in and getting up early for church made her grumpy. The Sunday dash was putting us all under pressure and when I weighed up the practicalities against the diminishing benefits to her, it was an easy decision to make.

Aileen and I agreed to continue taking turns each weekend, with a later start, and with a different focus. The chapter on church visits closed but we had other days out – Ian and I called them our 'Sunday Adventures'. We still spent time together and built on Mum's moments of happiness.

Chapter 10

'Resident's choice?': The Lonely Lounge

May 2013

The months rolled on and Mum still struggled to adjust to the day-to-day routine in the care home. It wasn't as I had imagined it either. Most residents, including Mum, seemed bored and spent a long time in the communal lounge doing very little. The cliché of the care home lounge with residents sitting dolefully around the perimeter of the room was now my mother's reality.

As an almost-daily visitor, I could see that the amount of activity on offer wasn't enough to keep residents stimulated. Occasionally there was an outing where four or five people went out but, other than that, nothing of any significance seemed to take place in the home.

As I arrived for my visits, I always prayed that there was something happening, and that Mum could take part. On the wall, opposite the lift, there was an activity planner that showed the plans for each day. As the lift doors opened, I checked for details, but they were often vague.

Keeping my tone optimistic, I'd ask 'What's on today on this floor?', but carers often looked skywards and shrugged their shoulders. There seemed no love lost between them and the activity coordinators.

Frequently, the words 'Resident's Choice' were written on the planner. This felt like shorthand for 'there's nothing planned' as I didn't see anything happening on those days. Even when each section of the board was fully completed, everyone knew that it did not reflect what happened in the home. Carers either ignored its existence or looked at it cynically, as if to say, 'that won't happen.' There seemed to be a grudging acceptance that the activity team weren't – excuse the pun – as active as they could be, and that nothing could be done about it. Things did improve, in some respects, a few years later but, back in 2013, life in the care home was bland.

I lost count of the times that residents who sat in the lounge said spontaneously, 'I'm bored.' Even those with poor memory asked for something to do. I wondered why these requests seemed to fall on deaf ears and why residents sat for much of the day facing the TV in the corner.

A regular alternative to 'Resident's Choice' was 'Movie Afternoon' – which meant a DVD of an old classic film. The explanation for this regular option came when I was informed 'They all love movies on this floor.' This seemed like a huge generalisation and – from what I saw – wasn't the case. For Mum, dementia had reduced her ability to concentrate, so she couldn't follow the plot of most TV programmes and quickly lost interest. I thought about this as I saw other residents not connected with whatever was on TV – movie or other. I had nothing against using films as an activity, but it felt like an easy option: passive and no different to the TV watching that went on all day, every day. Where was the variety?

The other problem with having a TV playing all day was that it stopped all conversation. As several residents had hearing difficulties, the volume was set permanently at high, making it virtually impossible to have a chat. For most people that would be a challenge but for those living with dementia, it created a bigger barrier and contributed to what I called 'the Lonely Lounge'. Dementia often negatively affects a person's social skills, especially if, like Mum, they have word-finding difficulties. Eventually, the verbal blunders affect their confidence, they retreat within themselves, and casual conversations disappear. As dementia progresses, even a formerly sociable person can lose their ability to strike up a conversation with someone sitting next to them. The result, in Mum's home, was a room full of people sitting around, wordlessly staring in front of them. The TV was constantly on with no one watching, while care staff went about their business.

Mum couldn't work out why everyone sat in silence, and no one spoke to her. She didn't understand and fretted about having 'no pals' there. Her usual sociable self didn't know how to fit in there, but she tried valiantly to make friends. I watched her shy smile as she offered friendly or witty comments and tried to catch someone's eye, only to be met with blank stares. *I* knew this wasn't personal – but *she* didn't. Others were in the same dementia boat. One day, I realised how lonely she must have felt when she stated, 'It would be better if I had a friend here.' My stomach lurched at the thought of my sweet, kind-hearted mother feeling so alone – and it was all happening in plain view of the care team.

The carers were hardworking and kind but seemed intent on getting their jobs done and getting through the routine of the day. They were always busy doing 'stuff,' but it seemed to go on *around* the residents rather than *with* them – apart from when administering any care task. There never seemed to be the time for carers to spend a few minutes chatting with residents and it made the atmosphere seem cold. Perhaps that wasn't built into their day – I wondered why on earth not – they weren't short-staffed. I couldn't understand why carers didn't take a moment, now and again, to encourage people to sit together and chat. Whenever I brought Mum into the lounge, I made a point of striking up conversations with other residents. I was surprised at how easy it was to get people chatting but could see that I had to keep pitching in to ease the conversation along. Instead, I watched as carers entered and left the room wordlessly.

Mum and I, in our separate ways, were perplexed by the disappointing reality of her life now. I thought: *Where' is the fun? Where is the laughter? Why does no one help them make friends? This is a nice home, but not a happy home.*

Again, I sought help from the manager, in the hope that she wanted to create a friendlier environment too. I tentatively suggested that Mum felt lonely and described what I'd observed in the lounge. Perhaps she needed a little help to give her the confidence to mix with others. Initially, the manager seemed sympathetic, before cautioning, '… but I can't force people to speak to your mum.' I could have slapped her.

'I don't want you to force *anyone* to do *anything*,' I smarted, 'but she does need your help.'

I left her office, exasperated that she didn't seem to see how she had a role in tackling the cause of Mum's unhappiness. At the time, I didn't know exactly what would work but I expected the care team to at least try. We continued with the Lonely Lounge.

If the idea of everyone sitting in a dull and boring lounge was frustrating, then the other scenario that Mum faced was nothing short of disturbing.

*****

Mrs B, the lady who often shouted at other residents, now dominated the lounge. She sat in the same chair each day and commanded the room with a stern voice, and sometimes with shouts. She often berated a poor soul for a perceived misdemeanour, and the staff seemed to accept that this was 'Mrs B's way'. Now and again, carers might pass a comment in her direction, but mostly they overlooked it. As a result, the lounge became a tense, edgy place where residents sat – presumably hoping that they weren't the target that day. I knew that this was part of Mrs B's dementia but felt uncomfortable that other residents were stuck in a tense atmosphere with nowhere else to sit. Technically that wasn't true, as there was another lounge on the same floor – the 'quiet lounge' – but this was used for storage and as a base for the activity coordinators. Realistically, residents had no alternative.

Mum learned, quickly, that the lounge wasn't a nice place to be, so she chose to stay in her bedroom. If invited there by a carer she might have agreed, not realising where she was being taken. Once in the lounge, she sensed the uncomfortable atmosphere and, after a few moments, made her way back out of the door. Carers helpfully obliged by returning her to her bedroom. Initially she was relieved to be in a quieter space but eventually she'd become restless which led to more confused thinking and, of course, worry. I was told that this cycle could be repeated a few times in any one day.

Avoiding the lounge meant that Mum wrongly developed a reputation as someone who 'prefers her own company.' I did a double take the first time I heard this and said, 'Mmm, I'm not sure she does,' but inside I bristled at their misjudgement. *That is not my mam's personality,* I thought, *she loves other people's company. It's because the lounge is horrible.*

Of course, I regularly talked about Mum's sociable side to anyone who would listen –but despite this they seemed not to question why she stayed out of the Lonely Lounge.

*****

After months of frustration with seeing how bored Mum and other residents were, I researched activity in care homes. There was limited information on offer, but I found a brilliant organisation called NAPA (National Association for Providers of Activities) that explained things clearly. It was like a lightbulb being switched on.

The problem seemed twofold and related to how the word 'activity' was perceived in the home. I've since learnt that this is similar in many care homes and needs to be resolved if residents are to live happy meaningful lives.

Firstly, what did they consider to be an 'activity'?

When Mum moved to the care home, I had assumed that it meant *entertainment* and I hoped to see a lively programme of events, games and hobbies. The vague activity board and the mundane life in the home showed me that little was happening on that front, but I didn't appreciate that there was a wider definition as well.

I discovered through NAPA and watching Mum and her fellow residents that meaningful activity could be *anything*. Some liked the social activities, while others enjoyed time alone doing low key tasks. Some preferred doing housework from days in their own homes, or using skills from their working life. It could also mean religious activity or keeping a link with the local community. It would be different for everybody but, with a life history document for each resident, they had the information they needed to make life interesting for them.

I realised that Mum's contentment did not depend solely on how much entertainment was on offer. Joining in with bingo or a sing-along might be enjoyable now and again but that did not give purpose to her day. Before she moved there, she was used to pottering around her flat engaged in little chores. Now she did nothing – not because she couldn't, but because everything was done *for* her. The kindness of the care staff had unintentionally meant that Mum and other residents endured long, boring days, without much to do. Yes, as we get older, many people want to slow down, or memory loss takes away some skills. But not completely and not to the point of living a dull life.

It seemed that no one at the care home had considered the deeper questions of: 'How does someone living here spend their day?' and 'How are they supported to do this?' I now pointedly asked myself these questions in relation to Mum.

The second part of the problem seemed linked to the first: thinking of activity only as entertainment. The grumbles I heard from carers hinted at this being a bigger obstacle to overcome.

Mum's home followed the traditional model of care staff focussing solely on care duties and dedicated coordinators organising activities. Busy carers saw how little happened in the home, and quietly blamed the activity team. They, understandably, felt that they had enough to do with their caring duties and did not see activities as part of their responsibilities. I remembered that previously I'd tried knitting with Mum and asked carers to prompt her when I wasn't there. They hadn't done it, but now I understood why – carers didn't think it was their job.

However, if activity meant 'how a person spends their day' then it was everybody's job to help. Carers, managers, family members could all play a part. I thought about how, in Mum's old flat, we had used household tasks to distract her when she was anxious – *they were activities*.

I researched other homes and learnt that several were moving towards a model of care where it was everybody's job to take part in meaningful activities. There, the whole staff team were explicitly directed, *and given the time*, to spend doing various things with residents as part of day-to-day care. This sounded ideal. However, at Mum's home they were nowhere near that point. There was a clear stand-off taking place; care staff – frustrated with the activity team – weren't going to do their job for them, and the activity team thought carers should be helping more.

It seemed obvious that they needed to meet in the middle. The activity coordinators needed to increase what they provided, and the care team could help with the simpler everyday activities. They could spend time reading, chatting, walking in the garden or helping residents to do little chores around the home. With a joint effort, residents could have a much more stimulating environment.

Now that I could see that part of the problem for Mum was the way the home viewed 'activity', I wanted to change that. I didn't know how to do anything about it yet, but at least I understood.

Chapter 11

'Where's Leo?': Separation

June 2013

Mum was missing Dad and couldn't fathom out where he was.

They'd been married for forty-three years when he died, and it hadn't been all been plain sailing. Our dad, Leo, was a remote and nervy man who was often angry and irritated by family life. He saw himself as a provider for the family and worked hard in the local shipyards. However, he also saw himself as 'the boss' of the home and we all hated his authoritarian style. Mum was the gentle one, who was generous with her smiles and cuddles, making us feel loved and cared for. She did everything 'for peace's sake' and smoothed out the bumps of family life even when we knew Dad was being unfair. That infuriated us. All three of his girls developed a keen sense of justice and didn't follow Mum's tactics as we grew into our teens and twenties. Rows with Dad were a regular occurrence in our house. I'm sure he felt outnumbered and was relieved when each of us left home when marriage, working away or a new life at the other side of the world called.

When Dad died in 2001, of course Mum grieved for her loss. After the initial shock and learning to live alone, I think she relished the freedom of being without her moody companion and enjoyed the more cheerful company of her friends. She lived a contented life as a widow but as dementia stripped her memory, by 2013 she had completely forgotten that he had died. When she moved into the care home, I noticed more 'Leo talk' and confusion about where he was. This was sometimes prompted by a photo of him but at other times it came unexpectedly. Perhaps with all the uncertainty she felt, her need for her husband's love and security was heightened.

On their wedding anniversary, I visited Mum and took their wedding album with me with the intention of reminiscing about their time together. I'd previously brought photos of Dad as he looked throughout their marriage and particularly as an old man. Mum's psychiatrist had suggested that this may prompt her to remember his later years … and eventual passing. That day she enjoyed looking through the album and we chatted happily about their lives together.

Later that same day, we were sitting in her bedroom and one of the male carers passed by the door. Mum spotted him and turned to me.

'I've just seen my husband,' she whispered. An expectant smile spread across her cheeks as if she hoped he would pass by again. She had seen the carer numerous times before, but that day, his thick dark hair must have reminded her of Dad as a young man. She seemed thrilled to have caught a glimpse of him. *She must miss him*, I thought, feeling wretched that I was about to dash her hopes.

'I think that's someone else, Mam,' I said, as gently as I could, 'but I know what you mean – he *does* look like Dad.'

I reached for one of the more recent photos of him on the wall and handed it to her.

'This is more like Dad,' I said, hoping something clicked and she'd remember this older, frailer husband and that reality would come back to her. I wondered whether showing her photos was a good idea, as it brought back memories and questions that I couldn't answer. I decided that reminiscing was a good thing and if that sometimes took her to a sad space, then I'd support her through it. We couldn't avoid every negative feeling.

By now, I knew not to tell Mum about Dad's death every time she asked about him, but I hadn't worked out how I should deal with it. It felt wrong to lie. My dilemma about deceiving her was resolved when another dementia support advisor caused me to consider the alternative.

'Can you imagine what it must feel like for your mam to learn about her husband's death as if it was the first time? Can you imagine her shock and upset if she hears this repeatedly?'

I saw things clearly from then on. I wasn't going to tell her he was dead ever again – gently or otherwise. Even though it felt uncomfortable, I settled on vague responses that didn't fully answer her question but avoided the crushing reality of his death.

One day when we were driving back to the care home after a short outing, she mused, 'I wonder what Leo has been doing whilst I've been out?' My heart sank.

'Oh, I'm sure Dad will be fine,' I said, nonchalantly. That seemed to satisfy her curiosity and I changed the course of the conversation.

However, over time she became preoccupied with his absence and the reason for her separation from him. 'Where's Leo?' was now a regular question. One morning in June we were in her room, and I realised the assumption she had made in her confusion.

'I think Leo has got someone else,' she said.

I was thrown by her words and plucked another vague response out of thin air. 'Oh, I don't think that could be the case, Mam.' I foolishly changed the topic without addressing her sad feelings. I was afraid to let her talk about him, so I chatted about practical things instead. It was a mistake, and a few days later she asked about him again – in a way that seared my heart.

I was at home, and it was early in the morning. The telephone rang, and by now I was accustomed to our morning calls. I prayed it wasn't a panicky one – it wasn't.

'Our Helen, I need to ask you something.' Her sweet and gentle voice made my heart burst with love for her.

'Yes, Mam, what is it?'

'I like the person I'm with here, but I love your dad and I want to be with him.' A new knot formed in my stomach. I was confused as to who she meant but didn't want to question her further.

'I know, Mam,'

'Have I been a good Mam?' she said. 'D'you think I'm a good wife?'

'Oh Mam, you are lovely, and we all love you!'

'I wonder,' she hesitated, 'if you see your dad, can you ask him if he wants to take me back?' Then doubt crept in – 'He might think he is better off without me.'

I thought my heart would break right then. I gulped back the tears.

'Oh, Mam, he is definitely not better off without you,' I said. 'I know he loves you, so let me see what we can do. Everything can get sorted. Shall we talk about it when I come up to see you?'

'Yes, can we?' Her voice sounded hopeful.

'I promise, Mam. Please do not worry though,' I said. 'I'll see you later'

I replaced the phone in its holder and slumped back onto the sofa. I ached to think of my loving mother imploring me to get a message to my long-dead dad and plead for him to 'take her back'. As we were growing up, she was the sweetest of women, keen to be loved and to live harmoniously with our grumpy dad. Even now in her confused state, she worried about what had gone wrong in the marriage and assumed that Dad's absence was because he had left her. Her vulnerability knocked me for six again, and I knew that my answers were only soothing her temporarily.

Later, I arrived at the home, but she made no mention of Dad. I was relieved but knew this tricky subject wasn't going away. Once again, I had fielded the 'Leo questions' as best I could, but they were becoming more frequent. There were times where in the space of one visit she repeatedly asked about him. What I didn't realise, at that time, was that her curiosity about his whereabouts was never going to be resolved until I gave her a satisfactory answer that soothed her emotions. I simply reacted to whatever she said, with no real plan of how to comfort her.

More worryingly, I had no idea what story the care staff were using when she asked them about Dad, and it hadn't even occurred to me to ask them. Later that week, I emailed my sisters to agree on a few phrases that might comfort or distract her. I thought we needed a consistent approach and used the term 'loving lies' but, even now, I have no idea where this came from. It felt wrong to be coldly planning to tell her any lies but that seemed preferable to upsetting her repeatedly. I also knew that we had to be specific in what we said. Mum still had a lot of insight at this stage, so using these 'loving lies' could make things worse. I ruled out my first attempts:

'Dad's out at the moment – but I know he loves you.'

'Dad's working away – but I know he loves you.'

I knew these were no good, as they had the potential to dig a deeper hole. I fretted over saying anything that forced us to tell a more elaborate tale to back up the original one. This all felt so wrong. I worried that she might remember that Dad was dead halfway through our tale and say – 'you said before that he was working away but I know he is dead!' Mum's dementia had made her doubt herself so much and she relied on us to help her understand things. Getting this wrong would have completely broken her trust in us. As sisters, we settled on a couple of phrases that we could use, depending on how worried she seemed. If she asked casually, we'd say, 'Can we have a chat about it tomorrow?' – hoping it might be forgotten later.

If she seemed more worried, we'd say, 'I haven't heard from Dad in a little while – but I know he loves you.' This was technically true. I hadn't heard from Dad, and I did believe that if there was 'another life', our dad would love Mum from wherever he was.

These felt like the best of a bad set of choices, so we went with them. As I studied more about dementia over the coming years, I learned that validating Mum's feelings of sadness by talking about how she missed Dad might have helped her more. I also learnt that term for lying to someone who has dementia, to prevent further harm, as 'Therapeutic Lies' – but all that came later. Back then, I went with the basics and what felt right. I was relieved at any minor successes and as these words started to give Mum comfort, I settled on them. But, as I had already discovered, with dementia, one set of worries is replaced by another.

*****

Mum had started to fret about her children – who were now in their fifties – imagining that she had to collect them from school. She also worried about her own, long-deceased, mum and dad, believing that they were poorly, and that she needed to look after them. These types of concerns are common for those living with dementia and later I learned that they can be a sign of an unmet emotional need. However, in 2013 I had no idea why dementia made her say these things.

Carers seemed to accept this as an inevitable part of dementia, but I couldn't write everything off as a symptom of the disease. I knew that life in this care home could be much better. I couldn't ignore the fact that I had seen her in situations where she was contented: at church, out with me and Ian, and at our house. I'd seen her smile, laugh, relax. I compared this with how she often appeared in the home – tense and anxious. She complained that she didn't know how to do things, didn't know what was expected of her in this new 'job', and, of course, that people didn't like her. Living in this care home was crushing her confidence. Once again, I agonised over how I could help her feel better.

We tried our best to visit most days but, as she couldn't remember the visits afterwards, she still missed her family. It seemed that, no matter how much time we spent with her, we couldn't fill that void. One afternoon, after spending a few hours together at a beachside café, we returned to the care home. I waved goodbye from the doorway of her room and was about to walk away when she said, 'Will I see you again?' It sounded like she thought I was leaving for good. My heart sank and my mind flashed to what she'd said the week before.

'If I could just see you a little bit more often, I'd feel better.' Poor Mum couldn't remember that within that same week I had visited on three other days and Aileen was there on the days in between. It seemed a hopeless situation; we couldn't do more, but it wasn't enough to make her feel still connected to us.

I churned the problem around in my head that evening. I realised that it was pointless expecting Mum to hold on to the memory of previous visits – this wasn't about facts – it was about a feeling. I had to find a way for her to know, if only in that moment, that I would be returning soon, and she didn't need to worry. She needed a feeling of security as I left her. On the following visit, I tried out my new way of saying goodbye that included a link to the next time I'd see her: 'Bye, Mam, Aileen is here tomorrow, and I'll be here on (insert day).'

'Okay,' she said, 'bye, pet!' her warm smile lighting up her face, with no hint of nerves.

It worked! I almost skipped towards the lift, immediately feeling lighter. I was relieved at this tiny bit of progress and made a mental note to use it after every visit. Of course, I knew that in a few hours she might forget the fact that I'd been there but hoped that the happy feelings associated with our time together would remain strong.

Chapter 12
'The Rita's Friends project': Another Plan
July 2013

In the summer, things suddenly took an upward turn. When Mum first moved into the home, I'd been told that there were regular outings, but I'd seen little evidence of them. Now, they were to be reinstated, with different residents invited on a rotation basis. Even if life in the Lonely Lounge continued to be dull, at least Mum would be going out now and again. Thrilled at this news, I let the activity team know that she was able to join in with most things – in those days, she could. Early signs were good when I heard that they went to a local social club for bingo, sing-alongs and coffee mornings. Then a visit to a local park, coffee shops and the seaside were planned – it sounded promising.

A few weeks later, Mum was selected to take part in regular sessions at a local community centre as part of an intergenerational project. Residents from a few care homes and one of the schools in the area were brought together for social activities. The thinking behind it was to help children understand dementia and to develop their kindness and empathy. It was a good learning opportunity for young people but also great for the residents too. They asked for volunteers to support the outings and I happily agreed to go along. Inside I was thinking, *Fantastic – this is just the sort of thing I had imagined for Mam when she moved here. Things are looking up.*

When I accompanied Mum to those sessions, I delighted at the change in her. Like on our church outings, she was transported from her worries and returned to her happy, sociable self. She loved mixing with the children, who had such a brilliant way with her and the other residents. They asked curious questions and listened intently to what the older people said, making them feel special and interesting. It was a joy to see.

After a few weeks, Mum was invited to take part in a video diary. One of the children was to interview her about her life and particularly what it was like when she was growing up. The coordinator asked if I had any photos that I could share so out came the memory book that I'd put together earlier from the contents of Mum's clutter bags.

On the day of the interview, I felt a tinge of nerves at whether she would be able to cope. While the main group took part in activities, Mum and I were ushered into a little room off the central corridor. Our interviewer, Alice, who was about eight years old, sat smiling on one side of the table with her list of questions. I guided Mum to a chair, opposite Alice, and perched next to her in case she needed help. As Alice confidently asked the questions Mum answered each of them, only briefly turning to me to check if she'd said the right thing. 'Yes, Mam, that's right.' I beamed with pride thinking, *she's doing so well.* Her grin told me she was enjoying the attention from the little girl, and I sighed with relief.

Afterwards, back in the main hall, Alice brought a few of her classmates over to meet us. She proudly introduced her new friend, Rita, and relayed snippets of what Mum had shared with her earlier. As they huddled around us, one boy asked if they could see the memory book they'd been told about. I thought I would burst – they were interested in my mum! The children stared wide-eyed, comparing the white-haired old lady before them with photos of her as a little girl, holding her favourite doll, and as a skinny teenager with friends. They giggled at the sight of her in a photo taken three years earlier, on the back of a Harley-Davidson trike in Sydney city centre. Mum visibly glowed as the children chatted away excitedly. I was on cloud nine. For me, it was further proof that, in the right situation, she could not only be calm but also happy. That day, I emailed my sisters to tell them what I'd seen and that I could see a way forward.

A few weeks later we saw the result of the interview in a charming DVD that showed photos of Mum in her younger days accompanied by Alice's voice-over narration. Again, she spoke of her friend, Rita, and it melted my heart.

*****

I was pleased with the new plans for outings but, behind the scenes, I was also working on getting Mum other companions to supplement our visits. If life inside the home was dull, then I was determined to find a way to brighten her days.

First, I contacted a befriending service for older people but was blindsided when, after an initial conversation with Mum, they deemed her 'not eligible' for their service. *Not eligible for a bloody friend!* I raged. *How can that be?* Despite their claims that they catered for those living with dementia, Mum's confusion – which at the time wasn't as bad as it got later – apparently meant that their befrienders were unlikely to have a meaningful conversation with her. I fumed at their rejection. *Isn't it about what Mum would find meaningful – not the befriender?* I seethed. Their lack of understanding of what dementia looked and felt like confirmed that they weren't right for Mum anyway – so I vowed to find our own befrienders. I had a new plan: the 'Rita's Friends' project.

I'd stayed in touch with a couple of ex-carers who had looked after Mum when she lived in the flat, and they came to visit on different days. One carer spent an hour or so having a cuppa in Mum's room and the other took her around the block in her wheelchair. Watching them laugh together as they reminisced about the funny things Mum had said or done in the past was heart-warming. The stories of her pulling funny faces or hiding illicit chocolate from her disapproving daughters made them giggle.

A much-loved niece, who had seen Mum regularly throughout the years, continued to visit. Mum had always enjoyed her company and I used to joke that she'd rather have had Christine as a daughter than any of us. My cousin's gentle, kind ways and talking about Mum's much-loved brother had kept the family connection strong. She always arrived with a beautiful bunch of flowers and a couple of scones for them to enjoy together. Food and good company – Mum was in her element.

Aileen enlisted the help of our friend and beautician, Stacey, whose regular visits brought a smile to Mum's day. Stacey had been doing Mum's treatments for years and we saw no reason why they shouldn't continue. Technically, the visits were appointments: chin waxing, manicures and the like, but the sight of Stacey's wide smile and friendly chatter meant so much more. Stacey loved Mum's sense of humour and, despite the sting of those waxing strips, Mum loved her in return.

I asked my husband, Ian, to visit one evening each week on the way home from work. He could see what I was trying to do so happily pitched in. They already had a great relationship and he still enjoyed teasing her in his gentle, harmless way. I imagined her face lighting up when she saw him, and on his return heard his tales of chatting with Mum and a group of other ladies. I think they liked his calm, soothing manner and – with very few men in the home – enjoyed the male company. I joked, 'I don't worry that my hubby is a bit of a ladies' man – he's an *old* ladies' man!'

I discovered that a friend from Mum's art class – some twenty-odd years before – now lived on the same street as the care home. She, and her daughter, visited Mum several times for a cuppa and a cake. Not long after the old friends had been reacquainted, the activity team invited people from the local community to join residents and relatives for Bingo once a week. Those same friends now became regulars at the home for what turned out to be a remarkably successful initiative.

The vicar from Mum's church popped in a couple of times in that first year and I tried to persuade other church friends to visit too. The response was lukewarm, and I felt I was having to push a little too hard, so I let it go. We were still seeing them on a Sunday at that point, so it didn't matter too much.

After the initial flurry, we hit a plateau and the Rita's Friends project eventually withered. The kind ex-carers soon stopped visiting as inevitably their lives moved on, and finding other people that Mum remembered was difficult. Lots of her well-established friends had died years before and others, who were still alive but ageing fast, found the journey to the care home too difficult. A few were young and mobile enough, but my not-so-subtle hints went unnoticed.

I didn't expect people to visit her every week or even every month, but I felt sad that Mum, who had been a good friend to so many, had little company now. I know people cared about her, but they couldn't find the time to visit, and they probably didn't realise how important it was. It had only recently dawned on me, in a way that I hadn't appreciated before, that spending time together is all we humans truly need. We all rush around, doing our own thing and catching up with family and friends only if time allows. Now I knew that, to someone living with dementia, those connections are much more significant. At a time when Mum felt disconnected from so much, I wanted her to feel loved and that she belonged.

At about this time, I read a blog from a daughter caring at home for her Mum who had dementia. She wrote, with fury, about the reasons that people gave for not visiting her mum. Excuses included: they 'didn't like to see her [mum] like this' or that it was 'too upsetting' (presumably for them). Of course, everyone is entitled to choose who they visit, whether in a care home or living independently, but I empathised with the blogger's anger. I had seen or heard other versions of this, including: not wanting to see the person with dementia distressed, wanting to remember them as they were (in happier times) and – the top prize goes to this – not feeling comfortable in the care home or when seeing other residents behaving oddly. By presenting these as noble 'excuses', some may think it is less hurtful. It is not. Fired up by the blog, I wrote my thoughts on this stance in my journal.

*****

Dementia is tough to witness. If I could avoid it, believe me, I would – but I can't.

I don't like seeing Mam in her distressed and confused state, nor do my husband or my sisters. Mam doesn't like being confused or feeling terrified and not knowing why – but she has to endure it. She needs us around her to make her feel loved and secure.

Mam is still a person with thoughts and feelings. When parts of our normal thinking are lost then we rely on feelings more. People need other people to make them feel whole. They need to feel the connection with the familiar – their old loves, lives and events. If we stay away, we are denying them all of this. We are isolating the person when they need us most.

For us, Rita was, and is, loved. She is valued now more than ever and will continue to be so, long after she is gone.

As for care homes – at first, they are bewildering for all of us. We didn't like the sights or sounds of care home life BUT we knew Mam needed to see us. We had to stay. We couldn't turn away and leave, even when we wanted to. Eventually care home life became normal and we grew to love and respect other residents as our friends.

So, if you feel you want to stay away from someone you love, who is living with dementia – give it another thought and give it another try. One day, that person might be me or it might be you.

*****

When I reread these words, they sounded indulgent and critical. I know it isn't my place to criticise another person's approach to dementia and how they deal with a loved one's illness. However, I can't sugar-coat my feelings on this and not comment on the other side of the coin. If we can't bear to *see* it, imagine what it must be like to *live* it.

I have witnessed personally and (later) professionally a person's enduring need for connection, and observed what happens when that is lost. I have encountered people forgotten by those they cared for and have seen the devastating effects.

I also thought about what I would want if I was living with dementia. I know that, from the core of my soul, the single most important thing for me would be that people do not forget me. Even when I forget who they are, what they mean to me and why we were connected, I would always want those people to actively be part of my life. I would need them to normalise the day-to-day life I have and help me find a reason to be happy each day. If every person that I know and love simply stayed away because it was too difficult for them to see me, then why would I be here? What would be the point of me living? This may sound dramatic but, for me, it is true.

So, I applied this thinking to my beautiful mum and dug in for the long haul. Rita's friendship circle may have gotten smaller, but we were no less committed.

I am writing this in 2022, when the world has endured more than two years of Covid-19, and care homes have been closed to relatives and friends for much of that time. That government-imposed separation had a catastrophic impact on the physical, cognitive and emotional wellbeing of thousands of residents. I advise anyone to read the newspaper articles from that time that describe individual stories of losses – and then decide whether regular visits matter or not.

Chapter 13

'Our little outings': Together in the Car

August 2013

I must have made hundreds of journeys in my car with Mum. In the early days, our trips were to hospitals, to church or morning outings that provided relief from the unhappiness Mum felt in the care home. We'd go to the seaside, and I'd ply her with ice cream – not the best choice for a diabetic, but it was a treat. Mum had routinely ignored her diabetes for years, so I risked an indulgence now and again.

Driving with Mum changed from being merely a practical task of getting from A to B to an opportunity for us to connect properly. My car was the place where we chatted, sang and laughed ourselves away from the claustrophobic world of locked doors and keypads of the home.

Despite her memory problems, Mum held a strong link between me and getting out and about. As soon as I arrived at the home, she assumed we would be off somewhere or other and heaved herself from her armchair. I was grateful that we managed to take her out so often and for so long, as other visitors told me their relatives had stopped wanting to go out. Not my mum – at any opportunity she had her coat on ready to join the adventures, and I was happy to oblige.

Mum's poor mobility made getting in and out the car a bit of a struggle, so I was relieved when Ian found a gadget to help. A brilliant tool that slotted into the car door frame when open and formed a handle that she could hold on to while she stepped inside. We had our routine down to a fine art. I'd stand behind her and prompt her by tapping the leg that she needed to lift first to step inside. 'Leg up, Mam – big leg in.' That was her cue to lift her leg a bit higher so she could step into the car. She'd then twist around so that she could get her bottom onto the seat and wriggle herself into a comfortable sitting position. Once settled, I placed a blanket around her knees as, like me, she was always cold. I'd reach inside to fix her seat belt, giving her a quick kiss as I stretched over her. I'd then heave the walking frame into the boot, and we were on our way. Journeys usually started or ended with a packet of Quavers. I had old-time music already cued up for the journey and we'd set off, singing our songs.

While I drove to our destination, I was constantly checking in on her. 'You okay, Mam?' 'You warm enough, Mam?' 'Are you happy, Mam?' When Ian was in the car with us, he said it was like a constant soundtrack in the background. It had become second nature and I hadn't realised I was doing it.

Mum would also be babbling away. She read out loud the words on the road signs as we went past them – 'No left turn,' then, further along, 'Roundabout ahead' – and, of course, the names of the places we passed en route.

Years later, the car was the perfect place for making our home videos. When Mum could no longer write, we stopped sending greetings cards to the family in Australia but recorded 'Happy Birthday' videos instead. Parked at our favourite spot, sitting in our seats with my phone positioned in a holder, we performed a rendition of 'Happy Birthday' to the lucky relative. Mum revelled in these performances and ad-libbed all the while. She added her witty one-liners and pulled funny faces into the camera.

As Mum's memory got progressively worse, the conversations in the car became more meaningful and often more poignant.

One morning, we were going for a day out and Mum said to me, 'Our Helen, will you teach me to do something?'

'Yes, Mam – what is it?'

'It's that thing you do. I've forgotten how.'

'What is it?'

'It's the thing you do in the shops.'

'What thing?'

'The thing in the shops where you get things.'

'Is it shopping, Mam? When you buy things? Do you want to learn how to go shopping, Mam?'

'Yes – that's it. I want to learn how to do that.'

It was an innocent enough request, but it made my heart squeeze. Anyone who knew Mum knew that she had always been a keen shopper. She loved to mooch around stores and bought trinkets and goodies to add to her already overloaded hoard. Later, when she was unable to get to the shops – resourceful as ever – she turned to catalogue shopping. Mum was a huge fan of mail order, well before the modern trend of online shopping. She subscribed to many brands and became a 'treasured customer' in no time. The piles of catalogues were stacked on her table in the flat and offered everything, from the household items you couldn't live without to ladies' fashion. She loved browsing through them and, of course, receiving the parcels. She even sought out a subscription to a high-end chocolate delivery service – despite the fact she was diabetic.

In the car that day, Mum was no doubt telling me that she missed the feeling of pleasure that shopping had brought her, and thought she'd forgotten how to do it. I resolved to take her to the shops to bring that happiness back into her life. Her poor mobility made it a wheelchair event, but we managed it a few times. On one shopping trip, she 'oohed' and 'aahed' as we made our way around the vibrant colours and multitude of styles – she clung on to a bright green scarf which we bought later.

Those conversations in the car helped me understand her thinking and, much further down the dementia line, a chat in the car brought a heart-warming moment.

Mostly, Mum knew that I was Helen – her daughter. Now and then she got muddled and asked if I was her sister or a friend, but mostly she knew our connection. In time, she would forget how she knew me, or my sisters, which I know devastated Aileen but, somehow, it didn't seem to bother me.

One day, we were returning from a routine podiatry appointment and were chatting generally about something or other as I drove us home. In response to something I'd said, Mum asked, 'What does your mam think?'

'My mam?' I paused and glanced at her.

'Yes.' I wasn't sure which way to go with this as I'd long since stopped correcting her on anything she said. That day she was in a good mood, so I gave her a straightforward reply.

'Well – *you* are my mam, Mam'

'What?'

'You are my mam.' I hoped that this wouldn't shake her grasp on reality and spoil the mood. It didn't – she beamed over at me.

'Am I? Well, I never! Well, I never!' she repeated.

'Is that okay, Mam?' I said, grinning from ear to ear. 'Is that a good thing?'

'Yes – it certainly is,' she smiled.

I beamed at her momentarily, and then returned my attention to the road ahead.

'I love you, Mam,' I said, a wave of tenderness washing over me for this agreeable old lady who was so loving even when she didn't remember our relationship. I didn't mind that she had forgotten that I was her daughter – but instead I marvelled at how easily she found contentment when she felt safe. She knew that she knew me, but didn't know how. I told Ian later, 'If she thinks she's got a friend called Helen – and she likes her – then that'll do for me.'

Those journeys together taught me so much and gave me treasured memories. The closeness inside the car and the fact that there were only the two of us (or three for Sunday Adventures) seemed to make communication easier for Mum. The conversations were simple and there were no other distractions, which helped her to focus. This became even more precious as Mum's words gradually disappeared.

*****

Some of our best times were in that car, but Mum hated returning to the care home. As we turned into the street leading to the home or approached the car park, Mum would realise that she was going back. It flummoxed me how she knew.

'Oh no! We're not going back there, are we?'

'It's okay, Mam, this is the new block of flats,' I'd say enthusiastically, even though her words gave me a sick feeling in the pit of my stomach.

The strange thing was that Mum was only jittery when walking towards the home and until she entered the lobby. Once inside, she walked, head down, concentrating on each step and admiring the tartan carpet. Passing the Manager's office, she was greeted warmly and, as she made her way to the lift, carers working on the ground floor called out 'Hello Rita.' She immediately felt welcomed, the fear faded and by the time we got into the lift, she was fine.

There were even glorious times where she arrived at the door to her bedroom, saw what must have become a familiar sight and said, 'I love this place.' My heart sang at hearing this, and it reinforced my belief that, despite the difficulties, staying here was the right thing to do. Mum had some positive associations with the home, her room and the kind staff there.

Nevertheless, those return journeys filled me with dread at the prospect of Mum being distressed, and I had to do something to fix it. I found a couple of solutions to distract her.

Once or twice, Mum had admired the few straggly shrubs on the path leading to the front door. So, in the springtime, I offered to buy new plants and spent one afternoon alongside my green-fingered mother filling the pots up with their new blooms. Mum's walk towards the home now became an opportunity to admire the flowers and distracted her from any jittery feelings. Years later, the home employed a great handy man who created more beautiful floral displays leading up to the entrance. *Perfect.* I was grateful for his thoughtfulness and thanked him countless times. His positive attitude was invaluable.

The other solution for us was to play a particular piece of music to distract Mum from her nervy feelings. We found the right tune completely by accident. One day, on the way to an appointment, I'd played a compilation CD of tunes from the past. Throughout the appointment she kept singing one song repeatedly and I wondered why she'd remembered that particular tune. I never did get an answer – but that was the day that 'Oh my darling, Clementine' became our happy song that we played and played and played. I used it when she was contented, when she was sad, anxious, and – if truth be told – when I had run out of ideas of how to cope.

*****

It wouldn't be a true account of our story if I didn't include the mistakes I made. Like other relatives who are catapulted into the world of dementia, I made my fair share of blunders in what I said and what I did.

Mum certainly let me know if I'd overstepped the mark in my caring role. If I'd gone too far in helping with something, or said too much, she'd say, 'Mamma, Dadda!' in a babyish voice, letting me know that she felt patronised. Or she'd stop stock-still, whatever she was doing, and say, 'Who is the mother here?' Suitably chastised, I'd step back into line. There were other bungles, too, that made us both laugh out loud.

One day, Mum and I were on the way out. We were running behind, even though the carers had her ready on time. As we stepped out of the lift and walked towards the front door, Mum announced, 'I need a wee.' My heart sank. I knew this would delay us, but I couldn't ignore it. I reassured her we were okay and hurried her into the downstairs loo. I flipped into toilet mode and got busy with what needed to be done. I was skilled at this and could turn things around in minutes. So I thought.

A few minutes later, in the car park, I reminded Mum of what she needed to do to get in the car. I tapped her right leg and said, 'Leg up, Mam – big leg in.' Right on cue she lifted her leg but stopped short. *Ugh,* I thought, *What's going on?* I repeated the prompt and she tried again. She still couldn't lift her leg any higher. 'What's wrong, Mam?' I said, and she tried a third time – without success. I worried that she was injured.

'Does it hurt, Mam?'

'No – it's stuck,' she said.

On further investigation I worked out what was amiss. In the rush to get in and out of the loo I'd pulled up her underwear but not her tights – the crotch of which was somewhere mid-thigh! No wonder she couldn't lift her leg properly. I knew we didn't have time to go back into the home so, to my shame, I stood behind her to protect her modesty and yanked those tights up to where they needed to be. It took less than five seconds to get her straight again and into the car – not a lesson in good care but a practical solution. I explained to Mum what I'd done, and we giggled all the way to the hospital.

*****

Our well-rehearsed car routine kept us going for years, despite Mum's physical and memory problems. Her willingness to hop into the car gave us the freedom to include her in our lives regularly and in several ways. Inevitably, though, we hit a snag as her dementia progressed.

One day in 2019, when we arrived at the clinic for her usual podiatry appointment, Mum refused to get out of the car. This was a new challenge for me, but I tried all my usual persuasion techniques: 'You need to have your feet looked at, Mam', 'The nurse is waiting for you' and, of course, 'I've got some Quavers for when we get inside, Mam'.

Mum bristled as she felt the cold from outside the car. 'No – I'm frightened. It's cold.'

I tried for a long while to reassure her, but nothing worked. It seemed that Mum had interpreted her cold feeling as fear and wouldn't budge. I cancelled the appointment. This was the start of another decline and, when Mum could no longer understand the usual 'Leg up, Mam' cue, I decided getting a wheelchair taxi would make things easier for her. Another phase ended and a new one began. I reasoned that we hadn't done too badly – we had enjoyed countless happy times in that car – now things were changing, and it was time to adapt again.

Chapter 14
'We are family': Residents, Family and Friends
September 2013

I constantly felt conflicted. The anxious phone calls were at their height, and told me of Mum's daily distress, yet care staff often insisted she was fine. I suppose they were used to seeing confused and upset residents and weren't as alarmed as we were. For me, the endless distressed calls didn't align with their account of Mum being okay, so I continued to worry.

To anyone on the outside, she *looked* fine. She was clean and presentable most days and staff were hardworking and kind. However, she hadn't settled there and, despite the hopeful signs earlier in the year, I felt the home didn't fully meet Mum's social, emotional or occupational needs.

I was baffled by a situation where routine boredom and loneliness were largely overlooked. About sixty people lived in this little community called a care home and around twenty of them lived on the same floor as Mum. Yet people seemed isolated. Yes, dementia had taken away aspects of their social skills, but there were carers around all day long who could have encouraged friendships and conversations.

I couldn't comprehend how Mum felt lonelier in a care home than she was in her flat – where she was alone all day except for us and the carers who came and went. Here, staff and other residents were around throughout the *whole* day, yet she seemed so alone. It seemed that a combination of busy staff, fixed daily routines and the culture of the home worked against having any real companionship between residents.

My heart ached for this kind, sweet woman who wanted what most of us want: to feel well, to feel loved, to be connected to others and to feel safe 'at home'. It wasn't too much to ask ... was it? Knowing this and doing something about it were two different things. I'd had a glimpse at the answer in my research, but in Mum's case, care home life was different to what I'd read. I knew that there must be a way for us to work with the care staff to keep her happy, but I couldn't force the issue.

I wondered what other relatives – whose loved ones had their own dementia struggles – thought about the home. I'd met quite a few over the previous months and some had become friends. Now and then, one might leak something in a conversation that indicated that they, too, were troubled by the dull atmosphere or other disappointments. We'd discreetly share grumbles about aspects of care while making drinks in the communal kitchen but, it seemed, we all had reservations about rocking the boat too much.

By then I had tentatively suggested loads of ideas for improvements, but most were met with a bemused smile or ignored completely. It felt like even the simplest suggestions were too difficult to implement and that I was getting on everyone's nerves. I felt like a lone voice and knew I needed support from others who also saw their loved ones' unhappy faces. I hoped that collectively we could make our voices heard. Of course, I continued to speak up about individual aspects of Mum's care, but I didn't want to be alone in my quest to make the care home better overall. Another plan was hatched: we needed a support network. *How about setting up a Family and Friends Group?* I knew not everyone would be interested but hoped that a few relatives would join us.

I initially mentioned it to one of the activity coordinators who, to her credit, was in favour of the idea. We took the suggestion to the manager, who agreed to try it out. I volunteered to get things started by writing letters to other relatives and roped Aileen into joining us. She went along with it on the basis that she wanted things to improve for Mum. I didn't want to be too pushy so started with the intention of seeing what others wanted from such a group. On reflection, I probably could have been more precise to avoid confusion about the group's purpose.

The first session was arranged. A few relatives attended and the entire activity team hosted the event. It was a tentative start, but we had several interested relatives and hoped to build on that. Over the next few years, support from the care home management was variable, but the activity team tried valiantly to make this group attractive to more relatives. They were great at arranging the meetings and welcoming those who attended. They tried so many ways to engage relatives that I felt sorry for them as the same old regulars trickled in. The emphasis shifted to more of a social gathering than a meeting, with wine and cheese on offer. That attracted a few new faces, but not many.

Each get-together saw the same handful of familiar faces, with perhaps the odd new addition. Although I'd found a couple of strong allies, who pitched up regularly, the response from other relatives was lukewarm. Some took the view that if there was anything wrong, they would talk to the manager directly – I agreed and did the same. Individual meetings could solve individual issues but what about the bigger picture? The Family and Friends group was to serve a different purpose: to discuss how general improvements could be made across the home. To my mind, everyone had a vested interest in the home but, for whatever reason, few had the appetite for getting involved in the group. I couldn't criticise or judge them as I knew how overwhelming care home life had become for me, but it didn't stop me feeling disillusioned. Perhaps it reflected the dynamics in the relationship between a care home and relatives ... but more of that later.

In the meetings themselves, the agenda seemed to fall into a fixed routine of the care team telling us what was going to happen that month (good), but little time spent on listening to the things we, the relatives, wanted to improve (not so good) and change was painfully slow.

I sometimes felt in the minority when expressing my views in these meetings, especially when I needed to raise the trickier topics. I spoke frequently about the lack of activity on Mum's floor and in one meeting this was met with surprised looks on staff faces. It baffled me as surely everyone – residents, relatives and staff alike – could see the yawning gaps and dull days. Sometimes, it felt like there was a glass wall between the relatives raising the issues and the staff on the other side.

On the way home from the meeting, I moaned to Ian. 'It's ridiculous! It's like *The Emperor's New Clothes*. Everyone acts like everything is okay and IT IS NOT! I'm sure it *is* fine if you've got all your marbles – but it certainly isn't if you are a bored, confused resident. They don't seem to get it! They don't want to hear the realities of residents' lives in their home.'

To be fair, there were some improvements that came about because of the Family and Friends group. Initially, there was no path in the large garden, but we requested a lovely walkway around the grass with raised beds. A few years later, the grotty kitchen area that had plagued me since Mum moved there was replaced with a clean and modern set up. However, the issue of the Lonely Lounge rumbled on without any dramatic improvement. I realised you could change the 'stuff' but might not change the culture as easily.

While the group did continue for several years, it lost direction and purpose. The months between the get-togethers increased and the attendance dwindled further. With hindsight, I wished that I'd been clearer on the intended purpose from the outset and that we'd had more ownership from the managers in our quest. Of course, I was grateful that we were allowed to set the group up at all, but felt an opportunity for something great was lost. In the almost seven years that Mum lived in that care home, there were four different managers in charge. Each of them approached the Family and Friends group in different ways, but I'm not sure that relatives were ever seen as 'partners in care'.

The lack of agreed purpose, the low uptake from relatives and the tensions didn't make for a sustainable model. Eventually, it fell by the wayside. The last Family and Friends get-together I attended in 2019 was a tense affair with two relatives (me and a newer recruit) and two members of staff. Hardly a group to champion change. After those difficult years, I was glad when it was finally over for me.

*****

However, back in September of 2013, away from the Family and Friends group, I was still battling to get Mum's personal care sorted. We had agreed a care plan, but the reality didn't always match the plan. In fact, it seemed that there were recurring problems that cropped up on rotation. On a practical level, it was frustrating but, more importantly, the inconsistencies were affecting Mum's day-to-day life.

Aileen and I regularly spoke with the Seniors, trying to resolve things informally. I kept my tone pleasant but was assertive about what had gone wrong. It seemed that, as one issue was corrected, another that had previously worked well fell off their radar without explanation. Aileen and I swapped notes, both exhausted at the effort it was taking to keep Mum's care on track. Having 'a word' with the Senior was happening so often that, I have no doubt, we annoyed them. We had no choice, though. Everything was on the plan for a reason and, when consistently applied, made a big difference to our very anxious mother.

Despite this, Aileen and I tried to stay positive, hoping that the glitches would be ironed out in time. I had heard stories of people taking a long while to settle into care homes and thought that our nervous mum must be in that category. Yes – these things niggled me, but I wanted to be fair to the staff. Carers were pleasant and in no way treated her badly but, when things were missed, it added to her discomfort and could lead to distress. I knew there needed to be a settling-in period and that mistakes would be made but, after a while, I started to doubt whether this was still a reasonable excuse. I needed to take this higher.

After the first meeting with the manager in the January, we agreed to meet regularly to discuss any issues. The routine became familiar even if the topic changed. The manager usually accepted the points I raised and promised to put things firmly back in place. Within days something went wrong. Perhaps a carer hadn't been told or didn't understand the change and then I'd have to explain the whole thing to them myself – all the while thinking, *this isn't my place!* I cringed as I was forced to remind the Senior of what had been agreed.

'I don't want to make a fuss but …'

'I've noticed that …'

'It's not a big deal but …,' I lied, wrestling with irritation and embarrassment. I reasoned that it was better to tackle it informally with the Senior rather than to go back, yet again, to the manager. It didn't matter – eventually things went awry again, and I was back at the manager's door. The inconsistency was the worst part. On any given day, whatever situation I encountered in the home either calmed me or made me want to scream – I never knew what each visit would bring.

'Nothing works,' I moaned to Ian one night, 'no matter what I say or do, we end up back at square one!' I was disillusioned with care home life and my hopes for Mum's happiness were crumbling.

Despite these feelings, I thought we had no choice but to carry on. Way back when Mum was first diagnosed, someone had told me that it was unwise to move someone living with dementia to a new and unfamiliar place. That information was firmly lodged in my brain so – once we had found what we thought was the right home – I thought we had to stay. We had made Mum's bed, she now had to lie in it.

Chapter 15

'The Lovely Rita': Try to Understand Her

October 2013

My mum still felt like a 'duck out of water' in this place. I couldn't understand it – Mum had always fitted in. Everyone who knew her described her as a 'lovely woman' and she even had the nickname – 'The Lovely Rita'. Yes, she was quite nervous because of her upbringing, but she'd always been quietly sociable.

Mum was born in 1931, the second child of our grandparents Hannah and Aaron. She was a timid and shy child. Living in wartime Britain was a frightening time for everyone, but Hannah was a nervous woman and prone to periods of mental ill health. As parents, they were loving and kind, but Mum was sometimes kept home from school to look after Grandma while Grandad went to work. Hannah, ever fearful of what might happen to her daughter, curtailed Mum's childhood activities while her older brother, Ron, appeared to have more freedom. Mum once told me that she resented the obvious unfairness and thought her cautious upbringing was the root of her own nervousness.

That, followed by marriage to a difficult, moody man and bringing up three lively girls, contributed to Mum battling her own depression. Those shaky emotional foundations, upon which dementia landed, intensified her anxiety. A doctor once told me that dementia could exaggerate an existing temperament – I saw that in Mum. This anxious lady, in this strange environment, surrounded by unfamiliar faces, became an anxious 'resident'.

After living there for months, I wondered whether staff understood her personality and what made her tick. Yes, her kind, sweet manner was hard to ignore, but other aspects of her character, temperament and individuality seemed to be examined time and again – particularly in the first year.

One day, while Mum was in the dining room, I looked through her care notes as I did every now and then. The manager had given me permission as it helped me understand how she was on the days I wasn't there. Inside the file, I found an envelope stuffed with scraps of paper, envelopes and cards – all containing notes in Mum's handwriting. As I read each slip of paper, my stomach flipped at the jumbled – but worried – words. A message on a shopping list pad read:

'Find Helen's Floor'

'Find Helen's floor otherwise I'll get on the first floor. Once again and loose track once again. Make track for the 2nd floor. Please – I'm her mam'

A lump formed in my throat, as I read the last sentence.

Other notes showed me she'd been scared. Heavy tears dripped onto my lap as I imagined how awful she must have felt when she wrote these. *Why were these in this file?* I thought. *Why haven't I been told about them?* I removed the whole envelope from the file, wiped my eyes and bounded towards the manager's office to ask those same questions.

The manager, for reasons best known to herself, immediately took a defensive tone. She explained that carers had, on various occasions, seen the notes around Mum's room and taken them to show her. She had instructed the carers to put them, and any others they found, in Mum's care file. The manager did seem concerned – but *not* about Mum's distress – about the note writing. I leapt to her defence.

'Mam has always written things down – she's done it for years,' I said. 'She's written poetry, letters and notes all her life so I'm not surprised that she's writing her thoughts out now.'

My mind flashed to happier times when she'd scribble notes on any piece of paper at hand. Most birthday cards she sent usually had a witty handwritten note or drawing somewhere on the front – we called it 'Rita Graffiti'.

To me, she was trying to capture her thoughts in case they were lost again.

'Actually, when Mam first started forgetting things, I specifically encouraged her to write things down,' I said. 'I've seen notes in her bedroom before but nothing like these, saying she's scared. Do we know when they were written?'

'No. I don't know,' she said.

I sensed, from her clipped tone, that she was looking for me to put a stop to the note writing, but I was having none of it.

'I'm not sure what I can do about this.' I stared, stony faced. 'I can't stop her and I don't want to. She's telling us she's worried.'

'I know, but it's difficult …' Her voice trailed off.

Difficult for who? I thought. *Mam is the one who is frightened!* Nevertheless, I needed the manager onside. 'I get that – but why don't we focus on what we can do to help her stop feeling so scared?'

'Yes – we'll keep an eye on things,' she offered, and I agreed to do the same.

I went home that day and, the more I thought about what I'd been told, the more I seethed. *How dare they keep that information from us? Do they think they're shielding us? I don't want to be shielded – I want to know the truth so I can help Mam.*

I hadn't told the manager that I'd found a bra a few weeks earlier with the words 'Help me please!' written in biro several times across the cups. Horrified at the sight of it, I took it home and sought Aileen and Ian's advice on what we should do about it. We had agreed not to mention it, but on seeing the collection of notes that day, things looked much worse. Obviously, there been more instances of distress – which staff had known about but not shared with me.

A few days later, after consulting my dementia support advisor, who agreed with my concerns, I was back in the office to set things straight. We eventually agreed a way forward to respect Mum's privacy. The carers weren't to read Mum's notes unless she asked them. Notes would not be taken from her bedroom unless she asked for them to be passed to us and they would alert us to any concerns. I was satisfied that the manager had put these rules in place, but it wasn't long before we had another 'little chat' about Mum's behaviour.

*****

It was hard to hear people talk about our mother in a way that didn't reflect the lovely, sweet old dear we knew. I sometimes imagined myself arguing furiously with them but, when it came to it, I had to be respectful and decent. It irked me that they scrutinised the things she said.

Some staff didn't seem to understand her sense of humour and how she used it to compensate for her lack of confidence. From pulling funny faces to rattling her false teeth (just like Grandad) she was always trying to get a giggle. She also came out with great witty quips. Sadly, her dementia meant that she didn't always get the context right or the read the mood of the room.

One morning, the manager alerted me that a member of staff had been offended when Mum joked, 'Are you going shoplifting?' as she left the room. I recognised this as something Mum used to say years before and I suppose we'd call it 'banter' these days. It was a harmless line that had become one of her go-to sentences when she struggled for something to say. I was crushed that they had taken offence.

Worse still, I discovered they had started keeping notes of things Mum said. I was incensed and immediately talked this latest revelation over with my dementia adviser. She, once again, talked me down from the edge, giving me some questions to ask the manager. *What was the purpose? Were the comments of every other resident living with dementia being logged? If not, why was Mam under extra scrutiny from the staff?*

Again, the response was vague: they would do this for any residents that they were concerned about – but no explanation of why that included Mum. I didn't like the inference. There was no hint of it being about helping Mum, to me it seemed they were moaning about an aspect of her personality that didn't fit their ideal. *This is a home full of people who say and do things that seem weird – they have dementia!* Mum wasn't odd, she was just being her playful self. I loved her because of the increased quirkiness dementia brought, not despite it. Surely they should do the same.

I respectfully asked for this extra focus to stop and for Mum to be allowed to express herself in a normal way. The manager agreed but warned that if anything did come up in the future, they would have to log it.

'Fine,' I said, 'let's deal with that if it happens.'

I'd heard lots of talk about personalised care, and their brochures gave the impression of 'living life your own way', but the reality was that Mum was expected to slot into their fixed routines and ways to live. No wonder she felt like a 'duck out of water'. I regularly felt that I had to justify Mum's actions, and their seemingly judgemental scrutiny of her stung.

Chapter 16

'A life of my own': Cutting Through the Dementia

November 2013

By now, most of Mum's phone calls were wrapped in a layer of confusion. Dementia and the panic she felt made her use the wrong words or get off track quickly, but all the calls had a familiar theme: being lost, in the wrong place or trapped in various locations. She often began the call with, 'I've made a mistake', then described the predicament she thought she'd got herself into and asked me to come to get her. Our makeshift phone/orange button routine gave her some reassurance that she was in the right place and should stay there for now. She had limited periods of relief, so I clung to those and believed that we were making progress.

By late summer, the panic and confusion were replaced by Mum saying that she didn't like the home or those she lived with. Her words wrenched at my heart when, one day, she said, 'I just want to get out and disappear. The day is sunny but inside I feel sadness. I want to walk in the sunshine. I want to be with a different group.' I was still to learn about 'unmet needs' but knew that at the core of her jumbled conversations she was unhappy there.

A few weeks later, in what was the most lucid conversation we'd had for months, she left me in no doubt. I was so struck by the clarity of her message that I made notes straight afterwards – I wanted to capture the strength of her feeling.

As soon as the phone rang, the familiar pang of worry stabbed at me. I looked to the caller display in the hope that it was a work call, but the number withheld message and the time of day indicated otherwise. I braced myself and answered with the cheery voice reserved for these calls. *I can't let her hear my fear.*

'Hello!' I chirped.

'Our Helen, is that you?' Her voice was urgent. Without waiting for an answer, she launched in. 'You've got to help me. I'm dreadfully unhappy.'

I knew that she'd had a rough couple of days as I'd had two calls the previous evening: one after teatime, worried that people didn't care about her, and another much stranger one that I couldn't understand. What I did know was that she felt anxious and needed reassuring. The churning feeling in my stomach intensified, but I tried to keep my voice soothing.

'What's troubling you, Mam?' This was my new tactic to get her to share how she felt. Sometimes just talking helped her.

'I'm really unhappy,' she said.

'Oh Mam, I'm sorry. What's wrong?'

'I don't know – I just feel terrible.'

'That's awful, Mam, but you know – you might feel better later today. You don't always feel like this. These feelings do pass.'

'I don't think so,' she said gloomily.

'You've had bad days before, Mam, and you always manage to come out of it. I think you might feel better if you have company this morning. Can you see anyone in the hallway?'

Clutching at straws, I tried to direct her towards finding a friendly face in the home. I wasn't trying to fob her off – it was true that Mum often felt better as the day progressed – but right now she needed someone to distract her.

Then, in what felt like a real moment of clarity, she said, 'I want a life of my own. I need to be busy and active – to feel different. If you are happy, it makes you a better person.'

I was shocked that she could articulate this so clearly.

'I don't want people to say, 'Oh, poor Rita, she's not very good today, is she?' I could clag them when I hear them say that. I don't want to be told what to do all the time – I want a life of my own.'

I assumed she was mimicking a carer, as I recognised the tone that a few staff adopted. Perhaps said out of kindness, some things sounded patronising or bossy and I knew Mum wouldn't like that. I smiled at her use of the Geordie word 'clag' to say she'd like to slap them when they used a pitying tone. She didn't want their pity, to feel helpless or controlled. I had seen enough in the care home by then to know that sometimes carers went too far in treating residents like patients.

Most carers were kind, but I had also witnessed a style, in some, that made me angry too. One or two talked about Mum as if she wasn't in the room and I had to make a point of including her in the discussion to remind them she needed to be involved. Others had a 'scolding' style of talking about what Mum had done or said that day and it took me all my strength not to tell them to 'sod off'.

'I know, Mam. It's really hard for you.'

'Helen – I want to be normal and to live a normal life. I want to be happy.'

Another pang in my tummy. I couldn't bear to hear her pain, yet I had to speak normally.

'What would make you happy, Mam?' I didn't expect a coherent answer, but she was quick to respond.

'A better environment.'

Wow – she's so clear. I was shocked that this marvellous woman, who mixed up her words every day, was able to cut through the dementia and tell me exactly how she felt. I couldn't disagree with her. From what I had seen of how she spent her days, life there was dull. Of course she wanted better.

Dementia then got the better of her. 'I'll go to school, and I'll be no bother.' She'd gone off course, but corrected herself again: 'I want to be a help to people. I want a purpose in life.'

I got it. She wanted to feel useful, and her life there was so limited. Our daily visits helped but there was still something missing – a feeling. What she said next was chilling.

'If you live like this you might as well be dead.'

'Oh, Mam! Don't say that! I promise, I will sort this out.' I was horrified at her words and thinking, *you've bloody got to sort this out,* yet I tried to sound optimistic. 'Tell you what, Mam, why don't we talk about it when I come up later today?'

'Do you promise?'

'Yes, Mam,' and with another of my pledges we said goodbye.

Tears pricked my eyes and shame drowned my thoughts. *For God's sake, Helen, your mam is battling through everything to make herself heard and get you to take notice of her. What else do you need to hear?* I knew this had gone on too long but – even worse – I knew I didn't have an immediate answer as to what to do next. I thought about the numerous meetings I'd had with the care home manager since Mum went to live there. *Had anything been resolved? – No.* My head was filled with contradictory, spiralling thoughts. It was like I was having an argument with myself.

What the hell am I going to do?	*You'll have to do more.*
I'll have to talk to the manager again.	*Why? It's pointless.*
Who else can I talk to?	*Nothing works!*
Why aren't we getting anywhere?	*You'll have to try harder.*
Is this still part of settling in?	*How much longer should you wait?*
What about finding another home?	*You can't do that – she has dementia.*
Would she be better off elsewhere?	*This home is nice; her room is comfortable and it's close to us.*

I leaped off the chair, desperate to do something right away. Then, knowing I was stuck and had been for a long, long time, I sat down again. My head in my hands, I wailed out my frustration. I was angry, I was scared and I was so incredibly sad for my mum.

The conversation on that November day wasn't the first or the last time she reached out to plead for my help. However, there was now no uncertainty for me. No matter what was going on in that home – real or imagined – I had to do more to fix this. Yes, dementia muddled things up, but she was telling me very clearly that she was still unhappy. I'd have to try harder.

Chapter 17

'The end of my tether': The End of the First Year

December 2013

We lurched on through care home life and somehow arrived at December. I reflected on the year that had passed and our list of things that were going wrong in cycles. Problems with how Mum was dressed, her diet and the home's inability to manage her incontinence all reared their heads regularly. Alongside that, the routine boredom that I believed was contributing to her anxiety hadn't improved. Other things about the way the home was run irritated me, but I had to overlook them and focus on Mum-related issues. When things went wrong, Seniors wrangled about who was on shift, why something was missed, or how busy they were – seldom focussing on finding a way to stop it happening again. That made me lose confidence in them.

I was exhausted, and I knew Aileen was too. 'I'm at the end of my tether,' I told Ian one evening, 'but I can't seem to fix this.'

Too scared to make a formal complaint – in case it led to more problems – but too disturbed by Mum's distress to leave things as they were, I was all over the place. I walked on eggshells one minute or bounded into the manager's office the next. I had informal chats and regular reviews with the manager but, after a year of trooping in and out of the office, I had lost faith in that process too.

I tried different approaches: smiley Helen, serious Helen, helpful, concerned, stern, angry, professional Helen. You name it; I tried different versions of myself to appeal to the manger, but regardless of what specific action was agreed, things regularly went awry. I'd find myself in the thick of it again, correcting carers about what needed to be done. What else could I do?

Of course, staff must have resented a mere relative telling them what to do and I sensed a growing tension. We all wanted the best for Mum, but we had different views on certain aspects of care.

Over the preceding year, I had absorbed myself in research about dementia and was soaking up new information. I attended a family carers' course run by the Alzheimer's Society and gained useful tips on how I could support Mum. I completed a Dementia Friends information session that introduced me to the concept of living well with dementia, and was so impressed that I applied to become a Dementia Friends Champion. My research on the benefits of meaningful activity in care homes spurred me on, too.

As I learnt more, I applied the concepts to Mum's care and was dumbfounded that only a few of the carers seemed interested in what might work for her. *Aren't the staff supposed to be trained in dementia care?* I asked myself. *Why don't they know this stuff?* I tried to give them the benefit of the doubt and suggested things informally and casually, but my opinions weren't always welcome, and some carers didn't hide their feelings.

One day, I'd been chatting to a couple of carers and had suggested something about Mum just as I was about to walk away. I took a step forward but, for some reason, glanced backwards – and caught sight of one of them rolling her eyes as if to say, 'Here she goes again.' She froze when she saw that I was still looking at her, but it was too late – I had seen it and we stood in an awkward silence. I glowed red with embarrassment at what felt like their collective contempt.

I knew I should have called her out but was so shocked that I didn't dare speak. Instead, I held their gaze until they walked away and then traipsed back to Mum's room. I closed the door, sat on her bed and closed my eyes. *Sod them,* I thought, sulking at their disregard for me.

Mum watched TV, oblivious to my mood. I shuffled along the bed until I was near to her chair and took her hand.

'I love you, Mam,' I said.

'I know, and I love you too.

'That's good.' I pecked her on the cheek, feeling the warmth of her approval – not like the carers beyond the door. Once again, I resolved, *I will keep going – whatever it takes and whatever they think of me.*

I was wounded by yet another example of their grudging attitude towards a relative's input and anything that deviated from their 'we are in charge' position. *They'd be happier if I'd just go away,* I thought. *Not a chance!*

I remembered a conversation I'd had with an experienced carer early on during Mum's time at the home. She'd said that she had seen the same pattern time and again; families brought their loved one into the home and visited regularly at first but, as the months rolled on, the visits became less frequent and then reduced to holidays and Christmas Day. I'm sure that carers took on the role of family for those residents, but I cheerfully assured her, 'Don't worry – we won't be doing that. We will be here 'til the end.' Now, I don't think they saw that as a bonus.

I respected the team's experience of caring for people living with dementia, but what they seemed to forget was: long before Rita was their 'resident', she was our mum. I had the benefit of knowing her personality, what made her comfortable and what made her uneasy. We needed to work together to support her, but they seemed so fixed in their ways. When things went wrong, we nit-picked about the detail, and it seemed that our views on what care should feel like were completely at odds.

We wanted our distressed mum to feel she could contact us at any time by phone; they didn't seem to want us to be disturbed by her. We wanted her to be encouraged to make friends; they assumed that she preferred her own company. We were concerned about the source of Mum's distressed behaviour; they attributed everything to a symptom of dementia. We tried to find workable solutions when problems arose; they appeared niggled by my suggestions. We wanted to be fully involved in decisions that were made; they seemed to resent our input. We tried to give honest feedback about the care; they took offence at any criticisms we made.

Day-to-day communication with carers was mostly friendly, but the approach to Mum's care felt like a 'them and us' situation, rather than 'partners in care.' Keeping the relationship cordial was exhausting. It irritated me that visiting Mum meant that I had to edit my natural self. I felt I had to maintain a 'smiley Helen' persona while hiding my frustration at the latest mistakes. I resented their scrutiny of our mum and what felt like disapproval of her family. We hadn't signed her up for this.

I longed for things to get better. Any signs of improvement gave me a bit of hope. I told myself daily, *things have got to get better.*

*****

With so many bumps in the road, a valid question would be, 'Why didn't you move your mum to another home?'

The truth is that, for the first year I, along with my sisters, was ignorant about dementia and how the care system worked. We were terrified to make a mistake of any sort that jeopardised Mum's wellbeing. It seemed that this was just the way care home life was, and we had to accept it. Even as my understanding about dementia care grew (along with the misgivings about the home), I clung to the belief that I could not move her – it would make her worse.

I also knew that this had the potential to be a great home and perfect for Mum. There were some residents who seemed settled there, so why couldn't we do that for Mum? She had a large comfortable homely room and staff seemed to warm to her. We liked them – they were nice – but they just couldn't get things right consistently. I deliberated endlessly whether it was better to try to improve things where she was rather than move her to a situation that could be worse.

Even then, my thoughts got stuck on *where else can she go?* I knew that, during the initial search, Aileen and I had visited several care homes and neither of us could see an alternative that might work for her.

So, with all those thoughts, I had committed to make this home the right choice for us. If settling in was going to take Mum a little longer, then we would keep putting one foot in front of the other until she was happy. I wouldn't give up.

Chapter 18
'Unmet Needs': Challenging or Distressed?
The 2nd Year – 2014

If learning is acquired through experience, then 2014 was a bumper learning year for all of us. The year started with a repeat of some of 2013. The worried phone calls, though harrowing to hear, convinced me that things were not right yet. Mum's perception of her situation may have been blurry but her ability to tell me how she felt was razor sharp. In a quest to get the manager to take notice of Mum's feelings, I fed her regular examples of the things she said – I had plenty.

The words that floored me while I was on holiday, talking to Mum on the phone: 'People don't care about me here. Someone said that Helen's not back yet but said it a cheeky offhand way. I'll be away from here and be no trouble to the people here. I'm feeling very unhappy.'

A few weeks later, she stated clearly: 'There's someone here I don't like. She gets on my nerves. She's very cheeky and I don't like her. I've tried, but I don't.' I didn't know whether she meant a member of staff or a fellow resident – it didn't matter – this was more evidence that she was unhappy.

I thought my ears would never recover from hearing my mum in such pain. One afternoon, again over the phone, she was clear about how this home was getting to her. 'I just want to leave the premises,' she said. 'I feel worn down with all of this. If I wasn't so exhausted, I would run away.'

'Oh, don't say that, Mam,' I said, 'it will get better.'

'But Helen – I'm afraid of the place now. It's alright talking and talking, back and forward but I need to leave here. This is a rotten firm, and I don't want this job.'

My stomach flipped when I heard those words. I had done all I could to check there was no danger there. I had turned up unexpectedly at different hours of the day and into the evenings to make sure that she was safe in their care. I felt guilty for even thinking that way as I liked the carers but couldn't dismiss my thoughts completely until I'd made sure. I'd seen the horrible cases of abuse in care on TV documentaries and, in the dead of the night, my mind wandered to *what if...?* Show me the relative who has never had that doubt – even if just for a minute. I knew in my heart she was safe, and Ian (Mr Reality Check) reassured me, 'I haven't seen anything that I would be worried about, Helen.' So, other than the inconsistencies in care and the terminal boredom – I was satisfied that she was safe there.

'Don't worry, Mam – I'll make sure it gets better.'

'So, I have to wait yet another day.' Without another word, she hung up.

The shame washed over me again. Despite her poor memory, she had become accustomed to my 'everything will be okay' lines. She was angry at my lack of action to get her out of there. She couldn't know that I'd been trying to 'fix things' for a year. Logic told me that she couldn't go to the mysterious 'home' that she longed for, but

I still felt I should do more to make her feel better where she was. In reality, I had tried everything.

The situation felt impossible. I was stuck – too scared for Mum to leave that home and too troubled at her staying. *What is going to happen if I can't sort this?* My imagination, fertile at the best of times, took me down a path of Mum being sedated, wandering zombie-like, and descending quickly to a sorry end.

The months talking to carers, senior staff and management didn't fix things in the long term. Yes, we had improvements for short periods, but it was inconsistent so the troubles soon returned. I worried that we were stuck in this loop forevermore. Some days, when I saw her tormented, I wondered if she'd be better off not being here at all. A horrible thought – but at least then she would be out of this misery.

An unexpected offer of outside help presented itself soon – sadly as a result of Mum's worsening distress.

*****

Up to this point, Mum's anguish was relatively contained. She wasn't a disruptive resident so, it seemed to me, that staff weren't overly concerned about her requests to leave or pleas for help. Unsurprisingly, as the situation didn't improve, Mum's response changed for the worse.

She still regularly packed her walking frame with her belongings, put her coat on and paced the corridors as if expecting to go home. She worried about where various relatives were and that she needed to be with them. On her floor, there was usually some poor soul or other, desperately searching for an exit and asking to 'go home'. I had seen them endlessly pressing the buttons on the security keypads that operated the lift, trying to work out the code so they could leave.

Whenever I saw this, my stomach tightened and I wondered if Mum did the same. The thought of it, even now, makes me claustrophobic.

While these words and actions are not unusual for those living with dementia, I now know that they are not inevitable. The family carers' course I'd attended helped me understand that the person is probably showing a need for love, comfort or security. That fit with our 'duck out of water' who, for many reasons, felt she didn't belong there. At the course, I learnt that it was best to try to respond to that need, but the carers at this home didn't seem to be doing that. From what I could see, their training on distressed behaviour didn't focus on tackling the reason for the distress – only on trying to distract people … something that I didn't see working successfully. They were always gentle and tried to persuade residents to stay but nobody seemed to question *why* they wanted to leave in the first place.

I know that carers must have found it difficult to watch people in distress and not know what to do but inevitably the repeated attempts to distract residents led to some unpleasant exchanges. It eventually happened with Mum.

One afternoon, the Senior told me that Mum had, the previous day, been particularly keen to leave, explaining that she had to collect her children from school. One of the carers suggested that she needed to stay there but Mum insisted that it was important that she collect her kids. This went back and forth for some time. The more they refused, I assume the more her frustration and worry must have grown. No doubt that worry escalated to panic, and she ended up insulting the carer.

Similar situations occurred a few times, and I understand that Mum's responses were confined to insults, swearing or telling the carer to 'shut up'. There were a couple of instances where she pushed an unwelcome hand away but there was no physical aggression involved – at that point. Afterwards the relevant paperwork was filled in, detailing each incident. I understood the need to record things but, when I read the notes, I winced at the accusatory tone they used about my mother. It didn't feel like they were recording the actions of someone who was ill.

This change in behaviour worried me and although I felt sorry for the carers, my focus was on what this meant for Mum. I soon found out.

One bright May morning, I was summoned to the manager's office where she told me that Mum's worsening behaviour was cause for concern and that she was being referred to a specialist team that dealt with challenging behaviour. I will use the term 'challenging behaviour' here, as that was how it was described to me back, then BUT I believe a more accurate description is 'distressed behaviour'. I'm pleased to say that more enlightened sources tend to use that term now.

Back in the office, my blood ran cold. *Shit! What the hell does that mean?* My brain tried to catch up with what I'd heard. Of course, I knew what challenging behaviour meant – but what did this referral mean? *Is this the start of them kicking her out?* The shock must have been written on my face because the manager quickly assured me that this would help Mum. She handed over a note with details of a specialist nurse who could explain the process further. I was to give them a call.

Driving home, I was devastated. My meek, gentle mum had been in such despair that she had lashed out, albeit verbally. I was afraid but I was also fuming. She was now labelled as having 'challenging behaviour' – like a naughty child. My poor mother had been communicating her distress to anyone who would listen for over a year. In my opinion, the environment she found herself in had exacerbated her problems, but now she was being referred to a specialist team to work out why she behaved badly.

To me, this was like denying someone food and then – when they are starving – referring them to a specialist to find out why. I drove home thinking about how messed up this system was.

The next day, nervous of what was to come, I rang the number I'd been given. The nurse explained the entire process and how it would help them understand Mum, what was causing the anxiety and her actions. Most importantly, they would put a plan in place for the care home team to follow. It made such good sense that I was immediately relieved and on board with the idea. *This is what we need,* I thought. *Maybe THEY can get the carers to do something positive for Mam.*

The first stage in the process was to complete a detailed life history document about Mum. I set to work, once again, logging everything I knew about my gentle, sensitive mother. However, this life history was different to those I'd completed in the previous year. The prompts and questions focussed more on her personality and her situation in the care home. I wrote about how she worried whether people liked her and was anxious in new company. How her nervousness and lack of confidence was masked by her quirky one-liners and jokes. How she was prone to low mood and depression but responded well to encouragement and praise. I shared the details of her creative nature and many hobbies. I wrote about her strong bond with her own mother, father and brother – a happy family unit – saddened later by her mum's long-standing mental health illness. She often said, 'my poor Mam'. Ironically, I was now using that same phrase about her. Another section asked about how she might react in certain situations; that's when everything suddenly became clear. It hit me like a punch in the stomach.

Laid out in front of me was a picture of my mum's personality and how she coped in different circumstances. When I compared this with the life she was living, I understood the impossible situation she'd been desperately trying to overcome. The expectation to fit in with this predetermined care home life was causing her intolerable stress.

The next section gave me a chance to describe the main problems from Mum's perspective. I focussed on three examples where Mum struggled and what I felt where the reasons that this created difficulties for staff.

- **Mum didn't feel at 'home.'** She didn't know that she lived in the care home, didn't feel she belonged there and, as a result, felt she was in the wrong place. This then led her to want to leave and to be frustrated at not being allowed to.

- **Mum didn't feel safe in the home.** She was afraid of some of the more vocal residents in the communal areas. She also feared for the wellbeing of others. As a result, she constantly needed reassurance that she was in the right place and was safe. When she still didn't feel safe, she wanted to leave.

- **Mum was bored and lonely.** She couldn't handle the noisy, intimidating lounge and so elected to stay in her room. This led to boredom, loneliness, confusion and eventually a feeling of being in the wrong place. She then wanted to leave.

Tears streamed down my face as I reviewed the information that I'd typed onto the form. This was a summary of an old lady's suffering – and that lady was my mum. The stark reality of what had been going wrong hit me full force. Of course, I already knew most of it. I had watched her live through each of these things individually – but now they all came crashing together. Dealing with her ailments and all the care home problems in the previous year had stopped me from linking everything into one clear picture. Now that I saw it laid out, I knew that her distressed behaviour was a perfectly logical reaction to the situation she perceived herself to be in.

As bleak as this looked, at least help was on its way. The next stage in the process was a meeting led by the specialist team to explore where things were going wrong. Aileen and I were invited, alongside the care staff from Mum's floor. A date was set the following month for the meeting, and I was raring to go.

*****

Everyone on the same page

On the allotted date, Aileen and I took our seats in the room that had been allocated for the meeting and waited for the others to arrive. My heart sank when I saw how few carers had turned up. I consoled myself with the hope that the deputy manager who was there would relay the information to the wider team. The meeting started with an explanation from the specialist nurse of how things worked, and I was keen to learn.

I heard about their model on distressed behaviour and how it applied it to my mum. They spoke of her 'unmet needs' and the 'triggers' that caused her to worry. I hadn't used those terms before but had suggested similar things. They identified the potential source of Mum's anxiety, anger and depression and highlighted how the environment had a big part to play. I thought about that lucid phone call and the numerous conversations we'd had. *Yes, Mam is painfully aware of the problems with this environment.*

I was then given a chart that summarised Mum's case and they worked through each section. I listened and made notes but no one else seemed to be doing the same – I wondered why. The nurse gave examples of the ways that Mum showed her distress: saying that she wanted to leave, packing her clothes, refusing food and, on occasions, making derogatory or insulting remarks. I pulled at the sides of my eyes to stop the tears falling as I imagined each scenario. I thought of what I'd like to say to the staff who logged these crimes. *Can't you see? Mam is distressed – not a bad person.*

Then we moved on to the insults that had brought her to the attention of this team. One entry showed an exchange where Mum had said she wanted to go home to see her mother and then (presumably when she was told she couldn't leave) said, '*You're horrible … you're a vicious slut.*' Aileen and I exchanged gloomy looks. Our mother didn't use language like this – she must have been distraught to say such a thing. Of course, I had sympathy for the carer on the receiving end of the insult but, if I'm honest, I thought more about Mum. She wasn't the first person I had seen distressed in that place, and I assumed wouldn't be the last. *Surely, they should have had training on how to deal with this.* I felt both apologetic and defensive at the same time.

There were more mixed emotions when the meeting ended. I was saddened to see the full picture of Mum's anguish but, having listened to the specialist's explanation, saw a way forward. I hoped that the carers now knew why Mum was so troubled.

A few days later a plan was drawn up which included some suggestions of how staff might use what they had learnt. The emphasis was on doing things to prevent Mum's anxiety taking hold, rather than waiting until she was already distressed and then reacting to it. *Proactive, not reactive – this makes sense.* The plan also stated that if Mum became distressed there was a sequence in which things should be done: first try to reassure her, if that didn't work then try to orientate her and if that didn't work try to distract her. Then – and only if these other options didn't soothe her – carers could utilise a 'Therapeutic Lie'.

This was another new term for me, but I could see similarities to the 'loving lies' that we'd agreed informally around Dad's whereabouts. I was relieved to see that there were some rules around using these carefully and according to the plan. Generic lies that casually misled Mum were not allowed – they had to be specific and only using the wording agreed. The manager and I worked on that aspect of the care plan. We outlined different scenarios and carefully constructed responses that we hoped would reassure Mum. Consistency was important. Once again, we focussed on keeping the responses as close as possible to reality without mentioning Mum's dementia or her relatives' deaths.

With everything in place, we just needed all staff updated on what had been agreed and then the plan could be implemented with Mum. *At last!* Relieved that we had something formal and tangible to help her, for the first time in a long while, I was optimistic.

Taking Action

The first few weeks went well. Carers got on board with the plan, Mum was less restless and made fewer panicky calls. We were going in the right direction.

Sadly, within a couple of months, things had slipped back. Mum was anxious again and the calls restarted. I rang the specialist nurse, who visited the home, checked Mum's notes and saw that staff input had petered out. They asked the manager to ensure that everyone reverted to what they had been doing during the first month when we had seen some improvement. They also referred Mum to an occupational therapist who provided advice on the types of activities that she could be involved in to prevent her distress.

Around that same time, Mum was officially discharged from the specialist team. I was anxious about being on our own without anyone checking what the home was doing. *How can we make this happen without their oversight?* Uneasy about the care home's erratic implementation, I wasn't convinced this would work.

The carers were good people – so what was going wrong? Once again – it seemed to be about communication. Most carers who worked with Mum hadn't been at the initial meeting, so they didn't have the full picture or grasp the significance of what we needed to do, and why. Over the course of several months, I repeatedly asked the deputy manager to share the information with her team but felt fobbed off when excuses followed apologies and reassurances came and went. From what I could see, the message still hadn't got through to the carers who needed it and Mum was still in turmoil. There seemed to be no sense of urgency on their part. It was now September and the action that we had agreed in July had not yet been implemented consistently. It seemed that because she wasn't high risk, they thought she could cope. I disagreed. Just because Mum wasn't tearing down curtains or climbing the walls it didn't mean she wasn't suffering badly.

I seethed: *How sodding scared does she have to be before they DO SOMETHING?*

The lack of action was one thing, but the ongoing lounge situation also compounded my worries. Mrs B, whose outbursts had worried me since Mum first arrived at the home, had gone into overdrive. She barked at both inanimate objects and fellow residents wherever she was. Every now and again, a brave soul would retaliate and an almighty argument would break out. Watching it was horrendous.

Having spent the last year learning about dementia and distressed behaviour, I realised that, on some level, Mrs B must also be distressed. I knew it wasn't my place to speak about another resident's care and my gentle prompts to staff fell on deaf ears. I wasn't complaining about Mrs B – that wouldn't be right – but I was concerned about the impact of one resident on many others.

I'd been conflicted about this for a long time, but the final straw came, for me, when one day I sat in the lounge, listening to the usual tirades. Mum inched closer to me and whispered, 'Just keep your mouth shut and then there's nothing to pick on.'

'It's okay, Mam – there's nothing to worry about,' I lied.

'But there is!' she replied.

Right then, I was jolted into the reality of the situation. My poor mother sensed danger but was permanently stuck between this mayhem and the loneliness of her bedroom.

Management sickness and holidays then meant further delays. I was livid and regularly chased it up with whoever was on duty. Feeling frustrated, one afternoon I marched into the office.

'Mam's care notes for yesterday show that she wasn't out of her room all day. How can we say we are following the plan?'

'Well, we can't force her out of her room,' came the response. I was reminded of the hurtful 'I can't force people to speak to your mum' comment from the manager the previous year. I couldn't believe that they had the solution to improve Mum's wellbeing right there and yet all they offered was glib statements.

'Mam can't do this on her own. We know what happens if she sits in that room all day. Your staff should have the skills to help her and there needs to be somewhere pleasant for her to sit,' I hissed. I wasn't usually that blunt, but I'd had my fill of waiting.

Once again, I was assured that something *was going to happen*, but I'd stopped listening – I'd heard it all before.

I tossed and turned in bed that night – sleep had become a luxury in those days – ruminating about the events of the preceding months. It seemed like madness. What was the point in requesting the expertise of a service that specialised in this area, who gave specific advice, only to fail at the implementation stage? Managers gave me different accounts of what carers were doing, but none of it matched what I was seeing. All the delays meant that Mum was still unsettled; she paced the corridors and continued to ask to go home.

Back to my food analogy. It was like starting to feed an undernourished person, rejoicing when they put on weight, only to stop feeding them and be puzzled as to why they lose weight again. *What are they thinking?* My fidgeting must have woken Ian, who checked to see if I was okay. I wasn't. I was at my wit's end and needed advice about what I could do about the mess we were in. I was desperate. I decided there and then, in the small hours of that morning, that I had no other choice but to contact the inspection authority in charge of care homes.

The very next day I made the call. My conversation with the inspector was meant to be purely to get advice, however, it set off a chain of events which took me down a route that I never intended. It triggered several conversations which shone a spotlight on the care home and made me more uneasy and unpopular.

It also instigated a meeting with a representative from the local authority, who agreed that the plans had not been fully implemented by the home – they asked that the specialist team return. The second meeting came and went with the same low attendance. When I complained, the deputy manager explained (almost apologetically) that staff weren't paid to attend that type of session so she couldn't force them. I now understood. *Why the hell should staff come in on their day off, unpaid, to do something related to their job?* I fumed that the organisation's policies didn't help the staff to help Mum. Over two meetings, only a handful of staff attended which left the remaining staff with no understanding of the finer detail that spelled out the problems.

Worst of all, we had invested another year in that home and now I didn't dare rock the boat by starting afresh anywhere else. I'd hoped that the specialist support would bring 'official' backing for helping Mum, which would resolve her problems. Yet, with the care home's patchy implementation, we had spent an entire year skirting around Mum's distress and had made little progress. I was sickened that the chance we'd been given had been frittered away.

*****

The reality was that, in the first two years, we were in constant turmoil. Writing these events here, they seem linear, but the living of it was frantic, chaotic and worrying. I was constantly firefighting against Mum's physical ailments and scheming for anything that improved her emotional wellbeing. There was no long-term plan on my part. With neither the time nor luxury of looking ahead, I dealt with whatever was in front of me.

2014 had left me emotionally battered and bruised. The realisation that we'd wasted a full year felt like a living nightmare where everything conspired against keeping Mum well.

I felt more stuck than ever, and Aileen and I fretted about what we could do. We constantly questioned whether we were doing the right thing. *Would anywhere else be better? Is this just 'the way it is'? At least they know her here.* We went round and round those questions and, with what we thought was no choice, clung to what we knew and any sign of hope.

Although I portrayed a strong, confident front – I was a mess. I gained two stones in weight and was comfort eating my way to a third. The extra bulk made me feel lethargic and lumpy - everything seemed like an effort. I couldn't sleep, and when not in the care home I curled up on the sofa trying to recoup the missed hours. My mind raced with everything that had gone wrong on any particular day and I endlessly replayed conversations I'd had with various staff members.

The repeated errors had made me lose confidence in the staff team, so I asked for extra checks to be put in place. I was hypervigilant and, eventually, even minor events became big issues in my mind. Ian helped me separate the significant errors from the inconsequential transgressions, but the latter still added to my concerns.

I cried, I ranted and raved. I was angry most of the time. If friends dared to try to defend anything about health and social care, that was my cue to launch into a tirade of accusations against the system. I was furious that other people could not see just how badly it was broken. Of course they couldn't – they weren't living through it – but Rita was, and so was I. In lighter moments I said I was suffering from CHSD: Care Home Stress Disorder. I was only half joking; it was making me ill.

Pleasant events were dulled by my low mood and my ever-present worry about Mum. On a sunny day, I could barely enjoy a day out without fretting that she might be stuck in her stifling hot room with no one to talk to. I couldn't stand it.

Finally, I went to see my GP and hoped I'd be referred for some Cognitive Behavioural Therapy. I was clear about what I wanted: support to help me deal with what I now realised was a tough situation that I couldn't fully control. I needed strategies to help me cope.

The first referral was a disaster as it was for those with Generalised Anxiety Disorder. My anxiety wasn't general at all – it was very specific, relating to what I had observed happening to Mum over the previous two years. The counsellor immediately recognised that I'd been misreferred, and sent me back to my GP.

The second was equally frustrating. The appointed counsellor spent most of each session telling me how difficult it was to work in the care sector. *I already know that!* I thought. *What I need is something to help me cope with the frustrations of care home life!*

The third referral was more promising. An eight-week course in mindfulness. I had read about this but, back in 2014, it wasn't as well-known as it is now. Nevertheless, I was happy to give it a go. I found the course interesting but ironically – with a head full of worry – found it difficult to concentrate on the technique. I'm happy to say it is a daily practice now.

I tried positive thinking, positive quotes, upbeat music – anything to keep me perky for when I had to visit Mum. I asked the universe for the care I wanted for her. I visualised her being happy. I prayed. I tried everything.

The only thing that made me feel any better was learning more about what Mum was going through and finding ways to help her. Knowing more made me feel empowered and less scared.

*****

Towards the end of the second year, the original manager left and the deputy took over her role. The first manager was a lovely warm person, who genuinely seemed to want to do the right thing. However, I couldn't ignore the fact that her good intentions didn't always translate to what the carers *actually did*, and that her plans hadn't stuck. The management change brought the prospect for a fresh start, and I prayed that a new regime would work. Secretly I wondered whether I was being an optimist or a fool.

With no alternatives available, once again I committed to this home. I would keep working with the new manager and find a way to make things better for Mum and her fellow residents. I would build on what we had started with Family and Friends, and work with the care team to make things better.

Some – including the staff – may have thought that it wasn't my place to try to change the home. Ordinarily I would have agreed. If Mum had been contented and comfortable for any significant amount of time, I would have happily shut my mouth and got on with my own life. But she wasn't – so I couldn't. I was now a daughter on a mission.

Part 2

A Daughter on a Mission

Chapter 19
Who Do You Think You Are?
2014

Loving, living and now, learning

God, I love this woman. As I sat next to Mum in her room, I thought about how things had changed between us. How much closer we were.

In my teens and twenties, I was frustrated by what I considered her lack of drive. Her 'anything for peace's sake' attitude at home drove me crazy. I saw her as weak, but I now appreciated that this amazing woman was anything *but* weak. She had endured numerous health issues throughout her life and now dementia dominated her world. Her resilience was remarkable.

Now, she was my first thought in the morning and the last one at night. My sisters were as puzzled by this transformation in me as I was, but it gave me a warm glow inside that our relationship had changed for the better. Seeing her face light up, as I walked in the room, filled my own heart with joy.

When I saw the struggles she experienced, living in the care home, I resolved that she wasn't going to live that way. I knew there were times when she was happy, and my aim was to keep stitching those moments together to make happy hours and days. When someone at church overdid the 'poor Rita' line too many times, I chirped 'she's not dead – she's got dementia – she can still have a happy life!'

Yes, this beautiful 'duck out of water' meant the world to me. Loving her and helping her live well in the home became my mission – it was all-consuming. My education now began in earnest.

*****

Learning

My learning started during those early conversations between me, a scared and bewildered daughter, and a helpful dementia support advisor. Our chats sparked my curiosity and created a ferocious interest in dementia. Each lesson delivered skilfully by the advisor helped me understand some of what it was like to live with the disease, from Mum's perspective. Those informal discussions taught me to stop correcting her when she made mistakes, or reminding her about Dad's death. I learned to go with the flow in all our conversations and that it was more important for her to feel okay, than for me to remind her of what she had forgotten. Ian must have found this change in me peculiar. I'd always had an annoying habit of pointing out any fact that he got wrong – however minor. Whenever we were with friends, he couldn't finish a tale without me butting in to correct him on the detail.

During those lengthy – often tearful – calls, the advisor calmed me down. She helped me order my jumbled thoughts and worries about Mum's care so that I could construct useful questions to ask back at the care home. Her guidance was a godsend.

Attending the Alzheimer's Society Family Carers course once a week towards the end of 2013 provided more valuable lessons, and I was Alzheimer's Society Family Carers course hooked. I learnt how someone living with dementia may be trying to communicate, and suddenly things fell into place about my mum. I learnt to look for the feeling behind Mum's words rather than focussing on the words themselves. The tutor explained that a person may be expressing a need for something else when they ask to go home or see their parent, or when they say they want to go to work. A request to go home may indicate a need to feel comfort or security, a plea for their parent a need for love or comfort, and stating they need to go to work might highlight a need for occupation or security.

Once I understood that, I wanted to share this revelation and couldn't wait to tell Aileen or the carers at the home. They must have thought I was a pain in the backside, but I was almost evangelical. I couldn't see any evidence that they already knew this stuff, so I brazenly told them.

I bought several books about dementia and spent hours researching details online. I discovered the things Mum did and said were far from odd – in fact, she was virtually a textbook case. I wanted to know more, and opportunities arose quickly.

Dementia Friends

In 2014, I became a Dementia Friends Champion – which meant that I trained as a volunteer to deliver information sessions to people in the local community. The sessions covered the five key things that everyone should know about dementia, with the aim of removing the stigma around the disease. This combined my two passions: training people and supporting people who were living with dementia. If I could help others understand what people like my mum were going through, then I would be making a small difference. It felt good to, at last, be doing something positive.

First, I learned about how language can affect people. Dementia Friends introduced me to the concept that Mum 'lives with' dementia, rather than 'suffers from' it – an expression which has such negative connotations. Yes, my mum *absolutely suffered* because of dementia, but the training helped me use words that promote a more positive outlook for her. I have used the 'lives with dementia' phrase ever since.

Next, I discovered the 'Bookcase Analogy' – a non-scientific explanation of how memory works. A video of the analogy can be found by doing an internet search of the words 'Dementia Friends Bookcase Analogy' but this is how it helped me understand the feelings side of living with dementia. I learned that the *feelings* a person has, about any given experience, will last longer than the *memory* of the facts. I'd seen this with Mum. She often felt bad about something but couldn't put her finger on what it was. Now I understood – the memory of the feeling had stayed, long after she was able to tell me what had happened. However, I realised that the same is true for positive feelings - they too last beyond the memory of the actual experience. The message, for me, was clear – I could help Mum by keep generating those positive feelings.

The training taught me so much that would have been invaluable at the start of our journey, and I was ready to spread the word. I started to deliver Dementia Friends sessions across the local community. I held sessions in church halls, supermarket staffrooms, community centres and other venues, but I also had my eye on one specific place – Mum's care home. I met with the Operations Director for the care company, who agreed that I could deliver sessions, not only for Mum's home but for homes across the group. Some sessions were for relatives, but others were for staff. I was delighted to be supplementing whatever training they already had with this more personal view of dementia. It was practical information that they could immediately put in place.

I'm sure some staff must have thought, *Who does she think she is – a relative, training us?* I felt a little awkward but powered on, hoping they would look past their scepticism and see that it could help residents.

*****

Care Home Managers

The previous year, I had attended a presentation from the local Healthwatch team and became interested in their work. Healthwatch is a national organisation, with a network of local groups, which gathers and champions the views of people who use health and social care services. They use this information to identify improvements and influence providers' plans, so I really liked the sound of them. I knew they were looking for volunteers, but wasn't sure whether the time was right to get involved. However, attending their event set off a chain reaction that ultimately changed the course of my career.

After the presentation, I shared some of Mum's story with one of the Healthwatch team. This led to several other meetings with her colleagues in the social care field, who asked for more detail. I told them about every bump in the road that Mum had faced since moving into the home. One particularly empathetic manager from the local authority invited me to present the main points to a group of care home managers at their next meeting. She thought it would be useful for them to hear things from a resident and relative's perspective.

'Could you give us, maybe, your top ten suggestions of how things could be improved?' she said.

Top ten? I thought. *I could give you my top thirty without even trying.* Grateful for the opportunity, I simply said, 'Yes – no problem,' and set to work on producing the list.

I was keen to share our story but was a little cautious about presenting the negative aspects in front of one person who I knew would be in the audience: the manager of Mum's care home. Regardless, I had to go for it. I anonymised the detail, so that the home couldn't be identified, but told the truth as we had experienced it. Each of the suggestions were rooted in something that had gone wrong.

On the day of the event, I arrived to find a large room filled with care home managers facing towards the front of the room where I was to stand later. My heart pounded in my chest. Even though I was an experienced trainer and facilitator, this was a personal story and, given the traumatic nature of the previous sixteen months, it still felt very raw. I hoped I wouldn't cry.

I found my place on a table near the back of the room, said a polite 'hello' to the woman next to me and waited for my slot on the agenda. The meeting began. The room was modern and had electric sockets fitted into boxes on the floor, covered with a flap that should have been flush with the carpet. Unfortunately, the socket nearest to me was missing its cover which, of course, I hadn't seen. As I listened intently to the person speaking, I adjusted my chair and as I did so, the leg dropped into the hole – making the chair tip backwards with me in it. I was flat on my back with my legs in the air! My neighbour rushed to help, and I scrambled to my feet faster than I have ever moved in my life. A few people turned when they heard the commotion, but I'd like to think that most didn't see the calamity happening. Later, still mortified, I referred to the mishap in my opening words.

'Good morning, I hoped that my presentation today would make a lasting impression on you … but perhaps not for the reason that you will now remember me.'

There were a few laughs, and I went on to deliver the presentation with what I hoped was a balance of 'daughter perspective' and professionalism. When I returned to my seat, my kind chair-rescuer smiled. 'Wow, and wow again!' she said, 'that was really powerful.' I hoped the others in the room felt the same and would consider what I'd shared when they went back to their own homes.

Afterwards, a few managers invited me to share the presentation directly with staff in their care homes. The sessions were well received, and the care teams seemed to appreciate my honesty. I knew things wouldn't change overnight but at least they'd heard how living in a care home might feel for residents and their families.

That was when the idea of working in social care first occurred to me. I enjoyed delivering the Dementia Friends sessions, had good training skills and was keen to do more. With my burgeoning interest in dementia care and first-hand experience as a relative – perhaps I had something to offer.

At around the same time, I became fascinated by the concept of providing meaningful activity in care homes. The potential to improve people's lives by focussing on how they spent their day excited me and gave me hope for Mum and her fellow residents. I was developing my understanding every day, and when the opportunity arose to study for a qualification in this area, I jumped at it.

Mum's care home manager generously allowed me to undertake training with a company that did their staff development. In return I offered to deliver some activity sessions in the home with groups of residents. They were simple activities like flower arranging, filling up bird feeders and some regular sing-along sessions, but they went down well with the residents. I loved spending time with the residents so much that I continued to do the odd session and also volunteered to help the activity team plan their programme. I was learning fast and there were lots of similarities that I could draw on from my decades in education. I had spent years running training centres and had good planning and facilitation skills. That, and my research about different approaches to dementia care, might be of some use to the team. I didn't want to seem arrogant, but I'd do anything to liven up the uninspiring activity planner that had plagued me for more than a year.

Of course, it didn't take a genius to work out my ulterior motive. If I helped improve what was on offer for all residents, then of course my mum benefitted too. I was more than happy to volunteer my services. The activity coordinators, understandably, had mixed feelings about my input. An extra pair of hands was always welcome, and I was happy to muck in with anything that needed doing. However, I was persistent about pushing for more activity on Mum's floor and I must have irritated them when my meddling brought into question how they spent their time. Who did I think I was?

I became so absorbed in care home life; it was taking up most of my time. When I wasn't visiting Mum and doing activities with her, I was working with the activity team. If I wasn't at the care home, I was planning something in my office. Every trip to the shops had me buying items that I could use with Mum or donate to the activity team. Ian joked, 'you do realise you have become your mam's personal activity coordinator?'

He was right. I hadn't intended to get this involved but once I got engrossed in care home life I jumped right in, feet first.

Chapter 20

The One-Woman Activity Centre

2014

Initially, whenever I visited Mum, I preferred to take her out as I thought that she spent enough time indoors. She was always keen to escape, and I was happy to provide a change of scene. However, after a while, I was concerned that she only seemed to be happy outside of the home – with Aileen or me. I wanted her to feel comfortable within the care home and that she belonged there. I started alternating my visits between us going out and staying home.

I'd asked countless staff to help Mum mix with the other residents, but it wasn't happening. Activity staff told me that most times, when they invited her to join the group activities, she politely declined. Of course, they took this refusal at face value. I knew that Mum often felt shy and needed extra encouragement to give her confidence. I had even made a note of this on one of the various information sheets I'd submitted earlier. No one seemed to make the link or question why she didn't join in. Oblivious, they respected her decision and moved on.

I wanted to build her confidence, so I joined her at the regular bingo sessions, or the monthly celebration events the home now had. These usually involved a large group of residents sitting in rows in the downstairs lounge, with a singer at the front belting out the old tunes. In fairness, when I was there Mum enjoyed these, but carers told me that she often left mid show if she didn't have a carer to sit by her side. That was Mum. Unless she felt safe and secure our 'duck out of water' took off.

After the distressed behaviour debacle in 2014, I was consoled by the fact that Mum now had an activity care plan drawn up by an occupational therapist. The message in it was clear – we should try to *prevent* Mum's distress by providing her with meaningful activities. The emphasis was on doing something before she got distressed as it would be harder to distract her once she became agitated.

When I read the plan, I smiled as I saw how it prescribed specific action that I'd known could work but failed to get in place for over two years. I had been like a broken record, but neither the activity team, the carers nor the Seniors seemed to understand the importance of what I was saying. I didn't feel smug; I was relieved that we had something official that staff could follow.

By now, I was regularly correcting anyone who reeled off the 'your mum likes her own company' line. The plan confirmed that Rita had been a social person in the past and that in the 'right social environment' she was 'contented and benefitted emotionally'.

I then read the specific recommendations and could relate them to what I'd seen.

- More one-to-one activity time rather than the big groups which caused her distress. *Yes – she can't cope with those big group events in the lounge.*

- Keeping small groups of people with a similar nature and ability level together. *Yes – she likes to sit with a small group of friends.*

- Having continuity of staff, who knew Mum, gave her a sense of confidence. *Yes! Mam thrives with the right, consistent support.*

The plan went on to explain elements of dementia care that I'd hoped the care team already knew but which I rarely saw in action. Particularly the fact that Mum (and others) needed support to sustain social interactions. I thought about the Lonely Lounge, with no one talking and an absence of staff input to initiate conversations.

I hoped that the plan, with its explicit instructions, would help them support Mum. With the manager's agreement I added some practical examples of activities that I knew Mum liked, and followed the suggestions. It didn't need to be complicated and it didn't need to take extra time – it just needed to follow the plan. We had everything we needed to try to prevent her distress. What could possibly go wrong?

*****

Activity in the home was marginally better than the previous two years but mainly consisted of larger group activities. Of course, that was better than the boring days of 'Resident's Choice' (which still appeared now and then) but the activities didn't appear to be personalised in any way.

Over time, I regularly reminded the activity coordinators about the suggestions on Mum's activity plan but rarely saw her being offered anything from it. There always seemed to be a reason to put things off. Staff sickness, changes in management and other issues all seemed to block Mum's route to a happier life. Frustrated with the lack of progress, I made my own arrangements and, as Ian had suggested, became Mum's unofficial personal activity coordinator.

I continued my research that I'd started in 2013 and looked for every opportunity to turn something basic into an activity for her. I discovered the term 'daily living tasks' and got Mum involved in those. If I brought her flowers – I'd turn that into flower arranging. If we were looking at her old ornaments – I'd turn that into polishing brass. We sorted out drawers, cleaned her makeup bag and dusted her room – all making her feel useful. We looked through catalogues and chose outfits that she might like – it didn't matter whether we bought them or not – it tapped into her love of shopping. I found a great reminiscence newspaper called, *Daily Sparkle*, and signed up for a free trial. Mum loved reading the articles and we chatted about whatever was in that day's edition. I thought it was so good that I suggested the care home got a subscription too.

Most visits, I tried to make sure we did something – just the two of us doing stuff in her room while music played in the background. I scoured shops for things that she might enjoy and arrived most days with a new item to explore or plans to resurrect the old ones. I tried anything to stave off the worries and keep her calm.

On the days when I arrived to find her struck with inexplicable fear and the need to 'go home', I'd suggest a change of scene. We paced the corridors together until she was happy to sit on a chair at the end of the hall and read a magazine or have a cup of tea. When that didn't work, and she bellowed, 'we have got to go! NOW!' – that was my cue to put on her coat and head out to the garden. We did circuits of the new paths, admiring the flowers, and I'd thank God that the Family and Friends group had persuaded the owner to have the paving laid. Other days we'd jump in the car, drive to the local shops for a bag of Quavers and, by the time we returned, the fear was forgotten.

As time progressed, I learnt that I sometimes needed to 'warm Mum up' to get her brain ready for an activity. Not a physical warm-up as such, but I'd repeat simple actions until she was ready to move on to what we intended to do. In my head, I worried about her skills slipping away: *you've got to do this now – you don't know how long she'll still be able to do it*. I concentrated on what she could still do and adapted activities to compensate for her failing memory.

The day that we first used Aquapaints was a revelation. Ever since the 'she can't put pen to paper' comment almost two years earlier, I'd tried different things to reawaken Mum's love for art, but so far nothing had worked. Aquapaints are sheets of card with images hidden underneath the white surface that are revealed when you use water to 'paint' onto the card. The impact on her was amazing.

That day, Mum was agitated and my reassurances weren't working. I had recently acquired a sample of the Aquapaint cards and thought, as nothing else was helping, I'd give it a try. I gathered the card, a paint brush and a pot of water, and placed them on the trolley table next to my troubled mum. I picked up the card and offered it to her.

'Look, Mam,' I said, 'see what I've found. Someone gave me this and I thought you'd like it.'

'What is it?' she scowled.

'Here – let me show you,' I said. 'It's something to paint.'

I put the card back on the tray table, dipped the brush in the water and then moved it across the page. The bright colours of a butterfly started to emerge.

'Isn't that brilliant, Mam?'

I knelt beside her and put the brush in her hand, guiding it towards the pot of water. After dipping it into the water, she moved the brush slowly across the card a few times. The outline of the butterfly and more colours appeared. She built up momentum, repeating the action and becoming more focussed with every stroke. After a few minutes, I glanced up. Her expression had changed from one of anger to sheer bliss. I could have cried. *It worked!* She had always loved painting, and this was a way she could do it now.

'This is great, Mam, isn't it? I enthused.

'Yes,' she said, smiling gently.

'That is beautiful. What pretty colours!'

'I know,' she nodded, as she continued with her task.

'That's it, Mum – you are doing great.' I urged her on, but I didn't need to. She was in her artist's groove and needed no further prompting. Her shoulders dropped as she relaxed and got deeper into the rhythm of painting. Brush in pot, brush on card, more of the image revealed itself … and so it went on.

All the while, I was thinking: *This is fantastic. It's changed her mood almost immediately.* As I kept watching her, it dawned on me that it was probably the brushing motion that reminded her of how she used to feel when she painted years ago. She didn't seem to notice the absence of real paints at all. Maybe the bright colours appealed to her as well, but that moment was a breakthrough for me. I realised it was about the feeling the activity gave her rather than the resulting picture. I remembered the Bookcase Analogy from Dementia Friends and thought, *my God, this could keep that happy feeling going for ages.*

I was like a proud parent and when one of the carers passed by the door, I called them into the room to show them Mum's masterpiece.

'Angie – look at this. Isn't it fantastic?' I hoped she would go along with my exaggerated enthusiasm for Mum's creation.

'That's lovely, Rita. What is it?'

I explained the idea of the cards.

'Like the kids' magic books?' she said. I hoped that Mum hadn't noticed that reference and thought it was a toy.

'Yes, but these are for adults,' I added quickly.

'That's lovely, Rita,' she smiled, and headed towards the door.

Later I saw the same carer in the communal kitchen and explained how the Aquapaints had transformed Mum's mood in a matter of minutes. She smiled back at me but seemed a little underwhelmed. I didn't mind, I was on a high and wanted more of this contentment for Mum. Using these could prevent the anxiety from appearing and soothe her for hours. As soon as I got home that day, I ordered more.

When they arrived, I created an art box with lots of paintbrushes and a collection of cards, which I left on a shelf in the wardrobe. I knew that Mum couldn't remember to use them of her own accord so I asked a carer if they could set things up now and again. After a few days, I saw no sign of the cards being used so I pinned them on Mum's noticeboard in her room and left it another week. I still couldn't see that they'd been touched but, on each of my visits, out came the art box. *Eventually they'll see how good they are.* Over the next few months, they became a regular pastime and were a godsend. They needed very little effort on my part because as soon as I prompted her, she happily took the brush and within minutes something clicked – she was in artist mode.

Fed up with wondering why carers still didn't get them out when I wasn't there, I decided to make them impossible to miss. One afternoon, when Mum went for lunch, I stayed behind and put all the equipment on the trolley table and wheeled it next to her armchair. *There we are – they just need to start Mam off,* I thought. As I left a few minutes later, I asked one of the carers to prompt Mum on her return and they promised they would. Success! She'd now have something to fill her afternoon.

Eventually, I regularly staged Mum's room with anything I thought she might like to do when she came back after lunch. I left magazines, catalogues, cuddly toys, balls of wool, or whatever else that might interest her, close to the armchair so that she could help herself to it when she returned.

Every little step in the right direction encouraged me to keep going.

*****

Healthwatch 2014

By 2014 I'd joined Healthwatch as a volunteer. One of their projects involved trained volunteers visiting care homes in the local area and giving feedback from a lay person's perspective. There was a specific framework to follow, but they were informal visits and focussed solely on the resident's experience.

I hoped that my knowledge of care home life as a relative would be useful to them. I didn't see myself as having all the answers, but I had more than two years' experience of what didn't work.

I underwent the training and soon started to visit local homes. I loved meeting residents, families and friends and interviewing them about their experience of care. I liked to think that, as someone who was close to their situation, I understood their perspective and was able to articulate their views accurately in my feedback.

I enjoyed seeing how other care homes operated and how practice differed between the homes. I hoped that our feedback gave the credit due for things that they did well and, where necessary, highlighted areas for improvement. I like to think I approached this work with a professional stance but, inevitably, the visits made me think about Mum. Whenever I visited a home that needed a lot of improvements, I felt gloomy about the sector in general. In homes that demonstrated great care, I was encouraged – if not a little envious – that the residents experienced better standards than in Mum's home. However, when I balanced out the pros and cons, I never left a home thinking, *I wish that she lived here.*

A common thread that ran through those visits was the importance of the people who worked there. What made the biggest difference to how residents and relatives felt about their care was the way individual staff members treated them. I'm sure that training and qualifications were relevant too, but the simple demonstration of kindness and compassion seemed to mean the most.

Chapter 21
Soft-Hearted: A Ray of Hope
2015

The one thing that I felt I could insist upon was Mum being up and dressed in the morning, with her hair brushed and makeup on. When she was first diagnosed with dementia, I saw photos of people with the disease that chilled my bones – old people, looking dishevelled and unkempt. I was determined that our mother was not going to disintegrate into a grey heap, and thankfully the manager agreed. It was a matter of retaining Rita's dignity – but for the first year or so, the results were mixed.

We were quite particular about Mum's hair. Aileen styled it on Saturdays, and we hoped the curls would last at least until the church outing the next day. Sometimes, we arrived to find a carer had unwittingly brushed the curls out and Mum's locks looked a frizzy mess, but usually they were intact.

Clothing was important too. Mum loved her clothes and accessories, so we made sure that she had a fully stocked wardrobe. We wanted her to look like her usual presentable self – and for days out, well-dressed. After frequently finding her clothes mismatched, I realised that good taste was subjective and that we couldn't criticise carers for not having the same sense of style. I didn't want staff to feel under pressure to find coordinating clothes for going out, so I prepared ready-made outfits in suit bags in her wardrobe and each week I restocked them from the clean laundry.

As toilet issues dominated our lives, we became preoccupied with Mum having a plentiful supply of underwear. The laundry service in the home was very efficient but she needed a LOT of stuff. I kept a particularly keen eye on the bra situation as I'd seen other ladies around the care home who clearly were braless, and it puzzled me. Of course, there could be many reasons why, but I witnessed it too often with various residents for me to think that it was always the individual's choice. I thought about how vulnerable I would feel without my bra when I was within sight of strangers. The oddity of care home life is that it straddles the concept of being a home as well as a communal living space for people who are unconnected to each other. In that situation – would so many women choose to be obviously braless? I'm not so sure.

For Rita, wearing a bra during the day was important on two counts. Firstly, my modest mother was never without a bra prior to dementia, and, in my view, we should respect that now. Secondly, there was the issue of physics. In 1989 Mum had breast cancer and a partial mastectomy. From then on, she had worn a breast prosthesis – we called it 'The Boob' – inside her bra.

One day when I visited her, she tried to explain that something wasn't right, but I couldn't work out what it was. I checked the usual toilet-related source but found no issues there, so we got on with our day. Much later, I was surprised to discover that a carer hadn't put her bra on. They'd put a thermal vest on and popped The Boob inside, but there was nothing to hold it in place. Poor Mum must have felt the silicone lump moving around, without being able to locate what was wrong or how to sort it out. She knew something wasn't right – she couldn't fathom it out. I could only imagine her frustration, walking around like that all morning. *What the hell was the carer thinking?*

It is fair to say that our attention on Mum's appearance featured heavily in our discussions with carers, Seniors and managers during the first two years. There were staff that understood the importance we placed on it, but others less so. When Kathy (not her real name) came to work at the home, everything changed.

Kathy was a young, smiley girl who quickly formed a bond with Mum, and I was relieved whenever she was on shift. She gave me hope. She took pride in establishing a morning routine for getting Mum ready that gave structure to her day. As Kathy helped Mum transform from her confused, dishevelled state after a night's sleep, into a well-groomed lady, the positive feelings began. For that small part of the day, the focus was solely on Mum, making her feel good and looking presentable to the world.

Although I wasn't there, Kathy told me of the chats they had between them. They discussed what Mum wanted to wear, which jewellery she wanted to put on, what Kathy had done the day before and other things going on around them. Music played along as they worked through the routine. *THAT is what good care looks like!* I thought. I meant no disrespect to those who had gone before her, but I had learnt enough to know that this gentle informal style worked successfully. Kathy's skill in turning this routine care task into a shared care activity (which Mum was actively involved in) made all the difference.

I saw how it helped orientate Mum towards the day ahead. Getting dressed helped her understand that it was morning time and that she needed to wear daytime clothes, not bedclothes. Assisting her to put her own makeup on must have given her a feeling of independence when there were so many other things that she could no longer do. Asking opinions, talking about life, smiling, and laughing together - all these are part of real relationships and everyday life. Kathy instinctively understood that the morning routine wasn't simply a care task to be gotten through as quickly as possible. It was a shared experience and Rita mattered. I knew that Mum would have sensed kindness and compassion during their time together.

The results were brilliant too. Whatever the day of the week, when Kathy got Mum ready, she looked great. Even when staying in, Mum wore the nice bright coloured clothes she preferred, had matching earrings and necklace, her hair was styled, and makeup completed the look. Whenever we went out, I'd arrive to find Mum resplendent with her hair in beautiful curls, looking neat and presentable. People we met often commented on how smart she looked. I'd beam with pride and couldn't wait to tell Kathy when we came back to the home. It wasn't about Mum being dressed up 'to the nines' – although I delighted in that – it was how it made Mum feel. It was no coincidence that on these mornings she also had a sunny, bright mood, and greeted me with the biggest of smiles and a 'Hello pet!'

Kathy wasn't the only one who did a great job with the morning routine – although she stood out. There were others who, with varying degrees of success, played their part in helping Mum start her day well. Aileen and I had a mental list of those carers we preferred to get Mum ready. Perhaps this was unfair. I knew that there were lots of reasons behind any successes but, as long as they tried, we were grateful for their efforts. I saw the difference between a good day and a bad day. A great morning routine usually meant that Mum looked well-groomed and was in a good mood. If things started well, we had a good chance of keeping Mum feeling good for longer that day.

On the other hand, if we found Mum looking bedraggled, forlorn, upset or – even worse, angry – I could usually trace it back to the morning routine. A bad start could easily extend to Mum having a bad day. It may have been something real or something she perceived, but the effect on her was considerable. It was hard to be precise about what had gone wrong, but sometimes I saw obvious clues. A few carers were a little gentler in their tone than others, some seemed too task-orientated and other subtle differences irked me. On those occasions, I felt irritated at the carer, but sometimes I could see it wasn't entirely their fault.

An unfamiliar carer from another floor might be sent in to get Mum ready without any knowledge of her routine and how important each element was. They may, with good intentions, have done the basics but invariably something was missed or left out. This left Mum feeling ill at ease and unable to explain what was wrong. I would arrive midmorning to find a raggedy version of my mum, with her mood equally raggedy. Sometimes she'd be crying, sometimes confused, agitated and, at worst, in a raging bad mood. On bad days she lashed out at all of us, greeting me or Aileen with a firm 'bugger off!'

I'd noticed several months earlier that she'd started to pick at a tiny dark blemish around her left eyebrow when she was anxious. This became a habit that would last for years – so much so that it eventually formed a large wart-like growth that sometimes bled.

I know no one intentionally did things to upset Mum, but now she relied purely on her feelings to determine whether a person was good or bad. Logic had little effect these days. If a carer seemed offhand or there was any jarring between them, she shut herself off from them to protect her feelings.

Mum wasn't weird or unusual in her need for a consistent morning routine – it was a matter of respecting her dignity. The topic of dignity is discussed a lot in care homes, with displays and statements galore, but I saw small violations many times which, to someone living with dementia, could upset them. Rather than the window-dressing of fancy posters, I wanted to see everyday examples that showed that staff understood and respected Mum's feelings. Some days I did, other days … not so much. A combination of busy carers, rigid home routines, staff shortages and a lack of effective training contributed to the more frustrating missteps.

But for most of the time, we were blessed with Kathy and her presence comforted not only Mum but me as well.

She completely changed how I felt about Mum's life in the care home. Knowing that this kind-hearted (she called it 'soft-hearted') person was there, and that Mum saw her smiley face throughout the day, reassured me. For the first time since Mum arrived at the home,

I felt that we were working as a team caring for her. Kathy told me when things were running low, or wearing out, or that another of her many necklaces had broken. She asked me to buy products that she thought made Mum's life easier such as the tee shirt bras instead of those with fiddly back fasteners. She relayed cute stories of things that Mum had said or done which gave me a better insight into how she was when I wasn't around. She was a naturally skilled carer with such a pleasant demeanour.

I frequently praised Kathy's morning routine to the Seniors and managers, in the hope that they replicated this with other staff and residents. I'm not sure that they fully understood that the point that I was making was about the impact on Mum's mood. In that situation, where many things weren't right, it seemed that whenever I praised good care it got lost in the noise about the negative stuff. I regularly complimented staff, but I wondered if they truly felt valued. I showed our appreciation in other ways too – buying treats for their afternoon breaks and other gifts that I thought they might like.

I tried to show Kathy how important she was to us. One day I took up a collage of photos that I'd taken over several months showing Mum looking her glamorous self. I was always taking photos of her, and we were doing selfies long before it became a popular thing. Mum loved looking at photos even though she didn't recognise herself as the person in the shot. She'd say, 'Oh she looks nice,' not realising it was her.

Before I put the collage on Mum's noticeboard, I showed Kathy.

'Do you see these photos of my mum looking beautiful, well-groomed and well cared for? I said. 'Well, these are the result of your hard work, and I really appreciate it.'

Kathy was, as usual, understated in her response, but I hoped that she knew that she was making a big difference to my mother's life. Other staff (they know who they are) did a great job too with the morning routine and, despite the other problems, I was grateful for this particularly consistent part of her care.

That was the difficulty for me. I was often conflicted by my warm feelings about the individual staff members and my mind-numbing frustration at the inconsistency in other areas of care. The twists and turns of the relationship between a relative and the care home were difficult to navigate.

*****

When Mum first moved into the care home, I encountered lots of experienced staff who were very knowledgeable. Some were efficient as well as pleasant, and I immediately took to them, but others seemed a little matron-like and, from what I saw, had an old-school approach to care. It made me feel uneasy and sometimes unwelcome in the home. As new carers were recruited, I saw a marked change in their style. Kathy and the others, with their gentle, upbeat characters made Mum happy. Mum's endearing personality made them very fond of her, but they had other residents to consider as well. Juggling the needs of several people with varying and complex conditions was difficult.

People working in social care are often seen in a negative light and their work viewed as unskilled. I never agreed with that view. I watched as I saw many of them juggle tasks and situations that I'm not sure I could have handled. They worked extremely hard and were always busy. I could see they were regularly under pressure and therefore needed to keep to a strict routine. That routine didn't allow any time for things to go wrong – as they often did, when dealing with people living with dementia. Mum's floor was the busiest in the home with a high number of residents who needed a lot of support. The ground floor had the same number of residents but many of them were more able and could do things for themselves. With a full house of complex needs, the staff on the first floor worked hard and must have been exhausted after their shifts.

I respected the carers and knew that most were doing their best. I saw them every day for several years and inevitably got to know them well. They shared stories about their personal lives as children and grandchildren were born. As I heard more of their news and views, I grew fond of them. We were connected by a common link – caring for The Lovely Rita. Of course, this made it so much more awkward when things went wrong. I worried that I was thought of as a tell-tale and making things difficult for them, but I had to do the right thing. My need for Mum to be well and happy was always greater than my need to be their friend but that didn't stop the knots forming in my stomach. They probably never knew that.

I also thought that the way the home was run sometimes contributed to the carers having a tough time – but what did I know about running a care home? Sometimes as an outsider, you can see things more clearly than those who are attached to their long-established ways. The more I learned about dementia the more I could see opportunities to do things differently. That might have seemed arrogant, but I didn't want to be the daughter who continually rocked up to tell them what had gone wrong. I wanted to help. I hoped that by introducing my little care hacks I could make life easier for them and Mum, but was disappointed when my suggestions fell on deaf ears.

I'm sure that all care homes aspire to have good relationships with their residents' families as it makes life easier for everyone. But to make that a reality, the care home team, who in my view hold all the power, need to view families as a help and not a hindrance. They need to make it explicit that relatives are valued as *partners in care* and encourage them to continue to be so. When it worked well at Mum's home – as with Kathy – it was heart-warming. When it didn't, it was soul-destroying.

Chapter 22

It's Not Just What You Do ...
It's How You Make Me Feel

2015

Even from the first year I was plotting to see how I could help –
not just with Mum, but across the home. Setting up the Family and
Friends group was my not-so-subtle attempt at improving things
along with other relatives. We did have some success, but it was
hard work. I moved on to running the odd activity session and
volunteering on projects with the activity team who now seemed to
have a love-hate response to my input.

Locally, there was an initiative being promoted in care homes across
the borough to introduce one-page profiles for each resident. The
one-page profile is a summary document detailing what is important
to the resident and notes on how they could be supported. I loved
the idea and quickly made a version for my mum and shared it with
the staff.

I volunteered to help introduce the profiles into Mum's home so,
with the manager's blessing, worked with the activity coordinators
on what we called the 'Getting to Know You' project. The idea was
that, if all staff got access to specific details about how the resident
might like to spend their day, they would know how to provide
meaningful activity. Again, while it was an aspiration for the wider
home, my motives were clear. I wanted this for my mum but, if other
residents benefitted too, I was more than happy to put in the work.

At the same time, my research led me to a resource called 'Make Every Moment Count' from the Scottish Care Inspectorate, which I incorporated into the project. It, like Dementia Friends, had five key messages for care teams – all aimed at everyone valuing the life of the person in care. The messages were:

- Get to know me

- **It's not just what you do ... it's how you make me feel**

- Know what I can do and support me to do it

- Help me feel comfortable, safe, and secure in my surroundings

- Remember little things all add up

The second statement on the list jumped out at me: *It's not just what you do ... it's how you make me feel.* I thought about Kathy and the others who had positively impacted on Mum. I also remembered when an offhand comment or clumsy approach set off the negative feelings.

Our project started with lots of enthusiasm and a flurry of activity. We managed to create profiles for many of the residents on Mum's floor, but later I was disappointed as their eagerness waned. Staff shortages, sickness and lack of backing from the management once again derailed our efforts and the project disintegrated. As a volunteer I had limited influence.

Healthwatch 2015

Away from Mum's home, I continued to do lots of volunteering work with Healthwatch and my endless chatter about meaningful activity had found some welcoming ears. The team at Healthwatch were very interested in how this impacted on resident wellbeing and in 2015 they made it the focus of their next round of care home visits. I could barely contain myself and, once again, threw myself into loads of work on the project.

This time around, our visits still focussed on interviewing residents, families and friends, but also included the activity coordinators in each home. Primarily, we wanted to know how residents spent their day. Once the visits were completed the data was collated and a report produced that provided some recommendations to the homes. The local authority – who had commissioned the work – were very supportive and included some criteria from the recommendations into their contracts the following year. Being so heavily involved in the project made me feel that, even as a volunteer, I was having an impact on care home life. This was to prove to be even more the case, the following year.

One of the recommendations in the Healthwatch report was to set up a network of activity coordinators in the area. I had plenty of experience of this type of work from my days in education when, between 2003 and 2011, I had facilitated a series of networks across the Northeast Region to develop teaching and learning techniques. I loved bringing people together to share ideas and now was keen to be involved with this new venture. At the same time, someone from the local care alliance was also keen to bring the activity coordinators together, so in partnership with Healthwatch we set up a local forum.

I knew that activity coordinators often felt isolated in their care homes. In 2015, the concept of meaningful activity didn't feature heavily on the priority list of many homes so training and development for coordinators was thin on the ground. The role was often seen as a 'nice to have', not a 'need to have', and as such some felt at the bottom of the pecking order. Often, fellow colleagues undervalued their work, thinking it was an easy job.

We invited activity coordinators from every home across the borough and developed a whole new community of practice. We based the learning content around the improvements set out in the Healthwatch report and things that activity coordinators themselves identified. Most importantly, this was a space where they could come together to share their experiences and ideas to develop their activity programmes. They provided each other with support and encouragement and stayed in touch with each other between sessions.

The activity coordinators I worked with were a dedicated bunch who oozed creativity and enthusiasm. Each session had a different theme and there would usually be some specific learning embedded into the session. We had guest speakers and arranged for them to visit each other's care homes to share good practice.

One of those visits was to a new, purpose-built specialist dementia care home, which had recently been built in the area. I'd met a manager from the company years before and they'd told me about their plans for the future. I couldn't wait to see this type of care in action and visited another home based on the same ethos, in Yorkshire. I was blown away by what was known as the 'Butterfly Approach' to care home life, with its smaller household-style living and a focus on truly person-centred care.

Now that we had one in our area, I wanted to show the activity coordinators how natural this style of care was and how staff teams could incorporate meaningful activity – not just entertainment – into everyday life. I knew they would be impressed by the shiny bright beautiful home but asked them to look beyond that, to see how some of the methods could be incorporated into their own homes. It was a great success, and the activity coordinators came back full of ideas and raring to go.

It would be a joy to work with this group for many years to come and I admired their determination to make life better for those they cared for.

Healthwatch 2016

By 2016 I was still volunteering with Healthwatch and when the next round of visits was being developed, I landed two roles. I continued to work as a volunteer visiting the homes but was also employed on a consultancy basis, to pull together the data and write the summary report. I was delighted at an opportunity to draw upon other skills that I hadn't used in a while and threw myself into that aspect of the work as well. Once again, the local authority incorporated our recommendations into subsequent contracts, which I felt was a great testimony to the work the entire team had put into the visits.

Dementia Friendly Communities

As a result of my ongoing work as a Dementia Friend Champion, I became involved in the local campaign for Dementia Friendly Communities. The Alzheimer's society definition was:

A Dementia Friendly Community can be a city, town, or village where people living with dementia are respected, understood, and supported to continue to live their life in the way they want.

I thought this was a worthwhile campaign and regularly attended the meetings. However, doing so brought home an uncomfortable truth that I'd started to notice during the years I'd immersed myself in care home life. In my view, the disparity was stark between what people *think* happens and the true lived experience.

Whenever a suggestion arose about how we could improve a person's life in the community, I was usually fully on board and tried to translate it to care homes. Each time I asked the question, 'What happens about this in care homes?', the same response was given. 'Care homes deal with that themselves', or 'care homes will already be doing this'. There seemed to be an assumption that care homes had everything fully in place, but this was far from the picture I was seeing in Mum's home and, by now, in other homes.

If the definition was *where people living with dementia are respected, understood, and supported to continue to live their life in the way they want* ... I could only conclude that, from my observations, care homes weren't truly Dementia Friendly – but everyone assumed they were. It was disheartening.

From my perspective, I'd been dissatisfied about the mediocre day-to-day existence Mum had, and often found myself thinking, *is this all we can expect from care homes in the future?* The more I learnt (both personally and professionally) from the residents and relatives I spoke to, I felt that things needed improving on a holistic scale. I loved everything I was doing but was also keen to be part of something further afield than Mum's home or the local homes – *could I work regionally and nationally?* I knew these were grand ideas but felt there must be some way for me to get involved. My answer came in 2016 when I found the Experts by Experience programme.

Experts by Experience

When I saw an advert for lay people to support the Care Quality Commission (CQC) Inspections, I leapt at the chance. Experts by Experience are people who have recent personal experience of using or caring for someone who uses health and social care services. CQC, and their partners, enlist those with this type of experience to support inspectors during an inspection. I applied and was thrilled when I was appointed on a casual contract.

The work was similar to the Healthwatch care home visits but followed the CQC inspection framework and was more formalised. I worked within my own region and sometimes beyond. Experts supported inspections by interviewing residents, relatives and friends to find out their thoughts and feelings about the care they received. Although still done in an informal manner, the interviews were aligned to formal criteria. At the end of each inspection, the Expert submitted a summary report to the inspector who would include relevant aspects into the final inspection report.

I enjoyed being part of this programme and contributing to the sector in a very tangible way. By now I was working full-time on all things care-home-related. I split my time between CQC inspections, running the Activity Coordinator Forum and Healthwatch projects. I was busier than ever.

As I learnt more about care home regulations, policies and procedures through this formal inspection structure, I kept coming back to my own mum's experiences. I was increasingly confused as to why, at her home, the system didn't seem to work quite as well as it was supposed to.

The reality was that, in my various roles, I'd heard countless similar stories from residents and relatives in homes locally and regionally. I saw my own frustrations paralleled in those people I met, who told me time and again of how they desperately tried to improve their (or their loved ones') care. Despite their best efforts, somehow the system seemed to be failing them. I knew the feeling well.

Chapter 23

A Fractured System – A Broken Spirit

2016

By the third year, Mum's home had improved in some respects. The change in management had helped but the biggest difference was in the staff. Most carers seemed to understand Mum's personality better and their warm smiles comforted her when she was nervous. I was relieved whenever they were on shift, and those who were less helpful were now in the minority.

I was reassured that Mum was a little calmer and I could see the positive impact of the morning routines. The distressed phone calls had reduced – although I sensed that this was partially down to her struggling to use the phone now. Instead, she soothed herself by pacing the corridors for what seemed like hours, chatting to staff along the way. Although they still hadn't mastered the concept of using meaningful activity to prevent Mum's distress, the kindness of the carers kept most of the panic at bay.

One of the very few blessings of Mum's advancing dementia was that she no longer had that feeling of being lost or in the wrong place so didn't have that agitated, unsettled feeling. I still felt that her care was inconsistent but there were some clear upsides to life for her now.

The downside, however, was that new things started to go wrong, and general standards were slipping. The communal areas of the home – which had always been free of any unpleasant smells – now had a distinct odour. As the lift doors opened onto the first floor I reeled as the smell of urine hit me. I politely pointed it out to carers or the Senior on duty that day, who called for the cleaner, but the smell would remain. Carpets were dirty and stained where once they had been clean. I found myself drawn into conversations as they justified their cleaning regime. *I don't care what you use!* I thought. *I just don't want the place to stink! My mum lives here!*

Staffing levels that had always seemed okay in the past now appeared to vary. On a good day there were the right number of staff – or I ought to say the number of carers that I was told should be on that floor. Even then, I could see that they didn't have a minute to themselves and rushed from place to place. On a bad day, they seemed to be firefighting, and I worried about how much time they had to notice – let alone respond to – residents' needs. I felt sorry for the carers, who shrugged their shoulders with a resigned 'this is how it is' look. Once, a carer discreetly suggested that I speak to the manager: 'It's the only way it will change, Helen – if families complain.' But, whenever I asked the manager, the cause seemed to vary – staff sickness, holidays, trouble recruiting. Things would improve for a while and then revert.

The biggest issue, for Mum, was that we were making little progress on managing her incontinence. To me, that meant having things in place to ensure she was kept comfortable, clean and dry. To be more specific, NOT (as I often found her) soaking wet with her clothes, chair and other items stained. Reasonable enough, I thought, and I suggested they tried prompting Mum to go to the toilet. By now Mum willingly accepted help from the carers so there was no issue with that, but we still seemed to struggle with a consistent approach. Every time one arrangement didn't have the desired effect, the manager and I tweaked the plans further, adding more detail. It went on and on. Ever-stricter regimes added further layers of complication to what I saw as a straightforward issue – and yet we still had the same problems. To say it was excessive was an understatement.

Staff were fed up and so was I. It seemed that tackling problems thoroughly in this home was impossible.

Informal concerns

My initial strategy of raising things informally with carers and Seniors had little impact as the issues relentlessly reappeared. I was torn. On one hand, the informal route wasn't working but, on the other, I worried about being thought of as overcritical. So, I decided on a different strategy: *If the same thing goes wrong three times, I will speak to the manager.*

I also redoubled my efforts in keeping accurate notes in the hope that if I gave the manager – let's call her Carol – precise details, she would have to acknowledge that these were not isolated events (which was the response I usually got). Perhaps, then, she would understand my utter frustration and find a way to make lasting changes.

One day, after a particularly bad experience the previous week, I met with the manager in her office to discuss what had happened. I wanted to explain things from Mum's perspective and how one mistake had a knock-on effect on the whole morning. As I walked into the office, she seemed to be dreading what I had to say. *Focus on the facts*, I told myself, *you're not making a fuss.*

I started with perhaps the source of the problem on that day. Despite the podiatry appointment being in the diary, the staff had 'forgotten' about it (or not checked the diary). When I arrived, Mum wasn't ready, and I had to dash around getting her dressed and rushing her to get to the clinic on time.

'She wasn't even properly dressed,' I said. 'She didn't have The Boob in, didn't have her slip on or the right stockings so that I could get them off easily at the clinic. I had to change half of her clothes. It was so stressful for her.'

She promised to sort it, but I wasn't finished. That was just the Rita stuff; I also needed to tell her about the problems in Mum's bedroom that same day.

'Her recliner chair smelt of urine, the protective sheet on her bed was missing and her mattress was wet. Mam would be mortified if she'd realised the state of her bedroom.' Carol knew that we had spent a fortune on various protective products to make life easier for carers and keep Mum comfortable.

'I promise, Helen. I'll speak to them,' she said, looking more serious.

'This is just one day's list, Carol. This is particularly bad – but we always have something or other going wrong. The topics change but the mistakes are similar.

I know the staff work hard and they care about Mam, but what can I do when I see all of this? I can't ignore the getting ready issue because it affects her day, and you know I won't ignore anything to do with her incontinence.'

Complaining – although I had cause to do it regularly – was not something I did lightly. I felt sick with worry every time I ended up perched on a chair in that office, but she didn't know that. She only saw the self-assured, confident daughter – not the jumble of my emotions. Feeling angry for being in that position again but pitying her at the same time. Feeling frustrated at the inconsistency of care but worried about carers getting into trouble and the impact on our relationship.

'D'you know that there are days when I sit in Mam's room and have to decide which of the mistakes I should raise with the carers or you? I feel as if I've got a limited number of complaint tokens and I must choose what to mention and what to leave out. It's not right.'

She was apologetic but I didn't want apologies, I wanted this complaint roundabout to stop and for her to get it fixed. I told her so. Nevertheless, she gave me more reassurances and with that the meeting ended.

As I trudged towards the lift to visit Mum, I choked back tears of frustration. Once the doors closed, I leant against the wall, head down, and shifted between the two versions of myself that I had created over the last three years: serious Helen and smiley Helen. One who was overwhelmed by the responsibility of doing the right thing for her mum. The other, who couldn't let anyone in this building know how crap she felt, so pasted a smile on her face for every visit. It was exhausting and that day I was deflated.

Only a few seconds to be myself, I thought, then the lift doors opened, and smiley Helen emerged. *Showtime!* I called 'good morning' to the carers and made my way to Mum's room.

I stood at the door for the couple of seconds it took for her to look up and spot me. 'Hello, Beautiful!' I said and she rewarded me with a dazzling smile. I walked towards her ready to plant a kiss on her soft cheek. *I can do this,* I told myself and pushed serious Helen away.

The energy it took to flip between the two different versions of me tired me out, but I never let her know that anything was amiss. She needed to feel safe and that, according to me, everything was okay. *I will make this okay, Mam.*

Looking back, I feel sorry for the Helen of that time who, despite three years of effort and disappointment still hoped for things to improve. I liked the manager and wanted this semiformal approach to work, but after a while I wasn't convinced.

*****

Formal Complaints

We continued to muddle along and despite my hopes for consistency of care under Carol's leadership – it was not to be. Things improved for a couple of weeks, or at best a couple of months, then they would revert. That was usually because they didn't tackle the root of most of the problems – poor communication. However, realising my limitations, I learnt to focus only on the things that directly affected Mum.

The myriad irritations about the way the home was run: the Lonely Lounge, the now-tatty furniture, and other gripes – I dealt with in other ways. However, the long-standing issue of how Mum's incontinence was managed did not improve. In fact, things were getting worse. Despite the various items we bought, the many care plans and the complex arrangements, it wasn't working.

Later that summer, I reluctantly decided to make a formal complaint. The details are convoluted, and not for disclosing publicly, but the way the process played out and the conclusions I drew about our experience in this care system were significant.

I checked the procedure fully and did everything required when sending the email outlining my concerns. I waited and waited – each week becoming more irritated by the lack of response. When the manager and I had other conversations, there was no mention of the complaint. I subtly checked that she had received the email and waited again. A frosty atmosphere developed when I was around the carers, and I believed that the manager's inaction allowed the problems to escalate. After a few weeks, I met with her again.

'Carol, I've not heard anything since my complaint email,' I said.

She seemed surprised that I was waiting for a formal response. 'Oh, I know,' she said.

'I think it's making things worse. I have to keep asking carers about what's going on [with my mum] and I'm sure they feel I'm on their case. They must be sick of me – but things are no better.' They clearly knew about the complaint and must have resented me going that far.

'Well ...' she said, hesitating, 'a couple of them have come to me.'

'What about?' I asked, sensing where this was going.

'Actually – about you.'

Oh no, I thought, *here we go – it's time to turn the tables on me again*. On a couple of previous occasions, after I'd raised a concern, I'd had to endure the indignity of listening to a one-sided, fuzzy account of what the staff thought of me. This time was equally vague about what I'd done wrong.

'What exactly do you mean?' I asked.

'Well, they *are* trying, Helen, but you don't seem to see that.'

'I do see that, Carol, and I appreciate all their efforts, but the facts I shared with you in my complaint show that things aren't right, are they?'

She couldn't argue with that, but added, 'I don't know. I've got staff complaining to me – saying that I'm listening to relatives too much.'

'*What?* I thought. *She is out of her depth.* However, I needed to reverse the direction of this conversation before it became all about me.

'I think we need to address the real issue at hand here – my mum's care – rather than turning the tables on me. If your staff do something wrong and I point it out, you shouldn't respond by telling me they have a problem with me. Especially as they don't have seem to have a problem until I raise an issue. Talk about shooting the messenger!'

Once again, I had that horrible mix of feelings that dealing with Mum's care triggered: anger, frustration and indignation on one side, fear and doubt on the other. It was hard to hear that the carers, who I saw every day, were criticising me – even though she couldn't tell me why. I'd worked hard, despite all the problems, to be kind and appreciative to the staff. I'd grown fond of them, but I couldn't overlook these problems. I felt insecure, hurt and vulnerable. *The old Helen wouldn't have felt like this*, I thought, *this is what this care home has done to me*. The relentlessness of the last few years had worn me down.

I stared at the desk as I considered what she'd said. I knew she was under pressure and, ironically, I felt sorry for her. However, I also expected a manager to be able to deal with her own staff dilemmas, but I sensed she'd merely placated them. She didn't know what to do, so she chose to turn the spotlight on me. Even then, she was painting an inaccurate picture.

'Carol, this just doesn't ring true,' I said. 'Yes, I'm sure they're pissed off with me about this complaint, but we get on well. We chat, we joke and talk about funny things that Mum has said. Surely, they wouldn't bother if they didn't feel we had a good relationship and that I appreciated them.'

'I know,' she agreed.

'Every time I leave this care home, I say 'thank you' to the carers on shift and I do it because I mean it. I know this isn't an easy job and I praise them for every little success. How many times do I come in here to tell you about something lovely that I've seen?'

I don't know why I'm pleading my case, but I do. I knew that even when I was burning with frustration, I made sure that the carers knew that I appreciated how hard they worked. This was not about individual carers, though; the way the home operated meant that things went wrong time and again. I refused to be cowed by this.

'What I won't do, though,' I said, 'is see something that is unacceptable and not flag it to the carer, the Senior or you. I have no choice.'

'No, I don't want you to do that. It's just … oh, I don't know.' I jumped in before she had a chance to say any more.

'They can't have it both ways, Carol. They can't say they like smiley Helen who praises them and buys them treats but then moan about her when she points out something isn't right. I am the same person, and it is up to you and your staff to do the right thing for Rita.'

Immediately, she flipped her stance as if I'd misunderstood the whole thing.

'Oh no, Helen, they think you are lovely and friendly. They know you appreciate them, but they are stressed out by this complaint and feel they're not doing their job properly.'

So … it's not about me not appreciating them. We now have the 'not doing their job' line. I was sick of hearing these clichés. I'd heard them before, and I wasn't going to get into that conversation again.

'Carol, I've said this before. It is not for me to judge whether your staff are doing their job properly. I am simply telling you what has or hasn't happened in this home and how it affects my mother. You must do something about it'

I hoped that I had put things back in the right order. She was the manager of the home; I was a relative who had made a formal complaint. We finished the meeting with me asking for her to formally respond to my email. She eventually did.

Despite my outward assertions I was bruised. As I left and walked across the car park, I heard chatting behind the fence as some staff were on their break. Given the conversation I'd had with the manager I imagined how they must bad-mouth me. No wonder I was on edge here – I always felt misrepresented, misquoted or misunderstood, so I overexplained things to compensate.

I knew that I'd done my best to give them the benefit of the doubt on so many occasions and see situations from their perspective – but when it came down to it, my mother's wellbeing trumped everything. I thought of the manager's response to a genuine complaint. *The bloody cheek of it*, I muttered to myself, *it's the same every time.*

A care home needs strong leadership for it to work well. A manager who understands how to balance the needs of the residents, the expectations of relatives and the challenges that staff face. That is a tough ask for anyone and I'm not sure, in their position, that I would get it right – yet I knew how it felt when they got it wrong.

I drove home fizzing with indignation at what I felt was her weak management style. Whatever the complaints procedure said happened, things didn't work like that. I ruminated on our conversation for days. I decided that there was an often used tactic when I (and others) asked too many questions, raised a concern, or a complaint. Their approach seemed to be deny, dilute or deflect the matter – all with an unspoken message.

Deny: 'No – that's not the case.' If I said something had happened (or not happened) they gave a different account. This occurred with small insignificant issues as well as the important ones.

Dilute: 'What's all the fuss about?' This was the next level and used when it was agreed that the problem had happened but, in their opinion, it wasn't as big a deal as I imagined. This could be by minimising the severity of what happened, the frequency (suggesting it was a one-off) or the impact on Mum.

Deflect: 'It is your fault.' When there seemed no other response available, the issue was ignored and I, the complainant, became the source of the problem. This was used whenever things got too difficult and, I presume, to weaken my case.

In all other scenarios, this would be considered unacceptable, but in this relationship, where all the power is with the care home, it seemed that relatives are fair game.

In my experience, the formal complaint process, and their commitment to change, was ineffective – but at least I had stood my ground. Over the years, there were several occasions like this. The account of events was distorted in favour of the organisation, or the carers, and I was painted in a negative light. Stories went back and forth, and I felt attacked and hurt time and again. When that happened, I clung on to the two mantras I had used that day:

'They can't have it both ways … I am the same person.'

'I am simply telling you what has happened. You must do something about it.'

Over the course of several years, I tried so many avenues to sort out my mother's care. Gentle comments turned into more robust requests; informal concerns turned into formal complaints. As each escalation fell on deaf ears, or nothing remedied the situation, there was no alternative but to turn to external bodies. Reviews with social workers felt like 'going through the motions' and didn't focus on how these errors must have felt from Mum's perspective. I grew tired of hearing the same lines: 'we can't expect things to be perfect.' *'Perfect' is far removed from what I expect these days!* I thought.

In other meetings, the facts I raised were glossed over or dismissed. More than once, I left with tears in my eyes and a feeling that they wanted 'issue resolved' stamped on the file. I felt demeaned and drained and vowed that I wouldn't put myself in that position again.

It seemed, by now, that I was thought of as a tell-tale by carers, a difficult relative by the managers and neurotic by some outside organisations. Those I complained to didn't seem to see the detail and the impact on Mum. I was left with an overwhelming fear that the wider care system did not protect Mum or me from any shortfall in standards.

I recognised that the problems weren't about neglect or abuse but, in my opinion, it didn't show an understanding of dignity in care and, in my mum's case, undermined the human experience. No one seemed to recognise that.

Who holds the power?

'Do you think I'm too picky?' I asked Ian, as he arrived home one day to find me lying, defeated, on the sofa. I gave him a blow-by-blow account of that day's events as he usually helped me rationalise things. 'Are my expectations too high?'

'No, not at all,' he said, 'you see what goes wrong and how it affects your mam.'

'Well, why doesn't anyone else see it?' I wailed. 'Why don't the carers think the stuff I raise is important? Why does the manager not sort it?' My arms were waving all over the place now as I lamented the unfairness of it all.

'Why do others – who are there to make sure everything works the right way – not see what I see?'

'I don't know. I can't understand it.'

'I feel like I'm in a different zone to them. The system doesn't work – no matter which way I look at it. I'm damned if I tackle the problems and Mam is damned if I don't.'

'Helen, I just don't know what to suggest,' he said. I hated it whenever he said that as it scared me that even my reliable rock of a husband didn't have a solution.

'The problem is that, as a relative, you feel all the emotional responsibility for your parent's wellbeing but have NO authority to make changes happen. This is a living nightmare!'

He still seemed stumped. I felt sorry for him, being married to me. I remembered our wedding vows a few years earlier and thought about the promise in the last line: 'Grow old along with me, for the best is yet to be.' *Poor sod*, I thought, *he has definitely been short-changed on that one*. Ever since our wedding day, we had been locked in this dementia and care home nightmare.

I knew I was delving into 'poor me' territory but I didn't care.

'What makes it worse is that I have to walk through that home every other day and know that they all have an opinion on me.'

'I know and it's not right.'

'The irony is that I am only in this shitty situation because Mam is ill. We can't look after her here, so we've got no choice but have her in a care home, but it's impossible to fix this.'

In any other situation that made me feel this bad, I knew I could do something to resolve it. If it were a job – I would resign. If it was with friends – I would opt out. If between me and Ian – I would leave. With Mum's care home, I didn't have that option. I was stuck in this relationship despite the feelings of dread it gave me. I felt panic at the prospect of no resolution and no way out.

Oddly, I still had the ever-present fear of her being kicked out of the home. Every time I raised any significant concern, at the back of my mind, I worried that Mum would be asked to leave because of me. I knew, from my work, that this was a common worry for relatives. The warning that was issued twenty-four days after Mum moved into the home had left its mark and the fear hadn't left me.

'I am literally trapped!' I wailed. 'I can't walk away, I can't accept the way things are and I can't, for the life of me, make it better. Am I doing this all wrong? They hold all the power and make me think that it's all my fault.'

'No – it's not you,' he assured me, 'this is NOT your fault.' He almost shouted the last bit. He'd had a ringside view of our plight and his forceful response made me feel marginally better.

I went back to comparing it with other scenarios. 'Actually, if this was a romantic relationship – there are laws against this sort of thing. You can't go around repeatedly telling people that their account of what happened is wrong. You can't question every issue they raise. You would be accused of emotional abuse.'

Something else occurred to me. I did an internet search on my phone and read it aloud.

'Gaslighting: The process of making somebody believe untrue things in order to control them, especially that they have imagined or been wrong about what has really happened.'[1]

'See what I mean?' I said to Ian. I may have been stretching the point, but this is how I felt. That I was the one being difficult, in the wrong and judged for something about my personality that I couldn't fix. Sometimes I wanted to run away from it all but I couldn't.

I knew that Aileen and Barbara supported me in principle and whenever we discussed an issue, they backed me wholeheartedly. However, with one of them living on the other side of the world and the other with full-time work commitments, I was alone in the trenches. I was the one who attended all the care reviews, raised the formal complaints, and wrestled the system. It felt lonely and scary – but I knew it would have been far worse if I hadn't had Ian by my side.

---

[1] *https://www.oxfordlearnersdictionaries.com/definition/english/gaslighting*

Chapter 24
Sunday Adventures: The Three Musketeers
2017

Dementia and care home life brought Mum a lot of sadness but there was also joy along the way. Her favourite times were Sunday mornings when Aileen and I took turns each week to take her out. For several years, this meant going to church, but when that stopped, Mum joined Ian and I on our Sunday Adventures. Every second week, Ian became my co-pilot on the 'keeping Mum happy' mission and together we negotiated each phase of her dementia – adapting as we went. We were 'The Three Musketeers'.

Sometimes we brought her to our house for Sunday lunch. There, she sat in a comfy armchair – a blanket covering her knees – glowing with contentment. She basked in the warm feeling of being with her family and doing normal things. Ian made lunch while we chatted about anything and everything. Usually, I had something to show her or something for us to do. I'd give her a *Daily Sparkle* magazine to read, which she did out loud, enjoying the sing-song rhythm of her own voice. She still loved reading long after she could comprehend the words or the meaning – it comforted her.

Sundays were also time for a Barbara catch up. Despite living several thousand miles away, Barbara stayed very involved in Mum's life. At first, she phoned regularly and when Mum could no longer hold the thread of a conversation, we switched to a Sunday morning *WhatsApp* call (usually in the car) or occasionally a *Skype* call at home. That way they could see each other, using smiles, waves, and short sentences so that Mum didn't get muddled.

Whenever she could, Barbara made the trip over to the UK – although expensive, it comforted her to see Mum for herself for a few weeks. I know it was torture for her to be so far away and unable to see her regularly.

One afternoon, I giggled as I walked into the conservatory and saw the set-up on the dining table. Ian had propped up the tablet, inside a large cardboard box to reduce the glare of the sun on the screen. He was always working out ways to help Mum and it worked a dream. I can still picture her peering inside the box while she chatted with Barbara, Simon and grandsons, Zebb and Eli.

Inevitably a trip to the loo was needed, which required all hands on deck to get her upstairs. Despite her poor mobility, stairs didn't seem to faze Mum too much – but to us they looked perilous. We were terrified that she'd fall so we created a 'Rita sandwich' with me in front guiding the way, Mum in the middle and Ian behind her in case she stumbled. We counted out loud as she went up each stair: 'one, two, three ...', encouraging her each time she heaved herself up to the next one. 'That's it. Well done, Mam!' The reverse journey was the same and we breathed a sigh of relief as we bundled her back into the armchair.

Sunday lunch was then served and Mum, with her healthy appetite, didn't disappoint. Slowly and steadily, she polished off the lot. Afterwards, a film and a sleep – like the old days at our family home in the 1970s.

We carried on for a few years until negotiating the stairs became too difficult for her. We tried using a commode downstairs but, by that stage, she was confused as to what to do with it, so it created more jitters. As before, we needed to adapt so we swapped to occasional Sunday lunches at a pub and other outings. It didn't stop the adventures.

We live in North East England and are lucky enough to have great beaches and coastal towns. As I drove along the seafront to our destination, Mum sat in the front seat of the car, her neck straining so she could take in as much of the view as possible. One morning, I think she was trying to tell us that she loved the sensation of whizzing along in the car but was so overwhelmed that she couldn't get all the words out. 'I just love it,' she kept repeating. I grinned at Ian in the rear-view mirror – her innocence melting my heart again.

The various seaside cafés gave us loads of different Mum memories. One, right next to the beach with its Robinson Crusoe castaway look, served huge scones that we ploughed our way through. Another, further along the coast, had a 1950s vibe and although it had a basic menu gave us great views of the sea. Further along still, there was a café that served fish and chips on one side and ice creams on the other. Double trouble – Mum was in heaven there. Across the road from the café there were some beach huts and once, while Barbara was visiting, we hired one for the day so Mum could be nearer the sea.

If we wanted a longer walk, the trusty wheelchair came out and we pushed her along the seafront promenade, as she pointed out the sights on the beach. One Sunday, we stopped at a skate park and Mum was thrilled to see the young people dashing backwards and forwards. 'Whey!' she shouted as each young acrobat made their way towards us. She was so full of delight for everything she saw.

Sometimes we'd visit parks and wheel her around the flower beds. She adored nature and pointed out each bloom as if it was the first one she'd ever seen. Garden centres, nature reserves, even walking among the raised planters in the care home garden, all made her happy.

A café at a local country park was one of her favourites. There was plenty of space, they served nice scones and had a roomy disabled access toilet. Ian and I were like a carefully choreographed team, one placing the order while the other looked after Mum. Whenever I returned to our table, I was touched by the sight of this little old dear and the love of my life with their heads together. Ian would be explaining something or showing her a photo on his phone while Mum listened intently.

A nearby lake had swans and geese. Once, after a short walk around the path, the swans surrounded Mum, hoping for food. Up close, they were far bigger and scarier than they appeared in the water, and I was a little concerned for her safety. She, of course, was oblivious, happily chatting away to them. I asked Ian to get between Mum and the swans – how very brave of me!

As her dementia progressed, so did the toilet fears – which cut short the amount of time we could be out of the care home. Later still, she became frailer and struggled to get in and out of the car too often. Undeterred, we adapted again and moved on to the next phase of the Sunday Adventures – we simply stayed in the car.

It was then that we introduced her to the delights of the McDonald's Drive Thru. Not for a burger, but for the joys of their hot chocolate in the winter and ice cream in the summer. She was particularly tickled by the notion of driving through to get the drinks and then driving off – with our freebies – not realising that Ian paid from the back seat.

No matter what we did – she embraced it all. Even when the adventures became very limited, she was grateful to be out and about. I loved seeing her like that and it spurred me on to keep finding ways to preserve those Sunday Adventures.

None of that would have been possible without the love and good grace of Ian. He gave up every other Sunday morning for years, to join the 'keeping Mum happy' mission. He was the third musketeer, my wingman, my second pair of hands (when I needed several) and my encouragement when things got tough.

He showed Mum love in so many ways. With his gentle comforting voice, he reassured her when she was uncertain. He chatted with her on any subject and seeing them together melted my heart. He teased her playfully and appealed to the joker in her. He knew how to adjust his conversation as Mum's dementia progressed, absorbing so much learning about the subject and how it might feel for her. He applied what he learnt diligently and focussed on keeping her happy. She loved him and felt safe in his company.

Unfortunately, it didn't always work out. On the odd occasion, Mum inexplicably turned against him for no reason and snarled 'just go away!' My gentle, kind husband took it on the chin and valiantly joined us two weeks later to do it all again.

Away from Mum, he comforted me when I paced our home like a wounded bear. He witnessed the sleepless nights, the endless tears, the rants and the rages. He was my confidant and my sounding board. He listened to my tirades against a broken care system and tried to help me navigate my way through it. He heard my doubts, my dilemmas, my fears and panic during the worst years. He encouraged every one of my schemes to introduce a new idea into the care home and accompanied me to all the fundraiser events they held. He endured it all. Without him I would have dissolved into a helpless mess.

We had been together for over fifteen years before Mum became ill and I loved him dearly. However, seeing him with her during those difficult years and feeling his unending support for me made me love him even more. I could not have done any of this without him by my side.

*****

Daily Sparkle

In 2017, another substantial change came along. I saw an advert for a role with the company who produced the *Daily Sparkle* to deliver their activity coordinator training. I'd been using their reminiscence newspapers on and off for years with Mum and she enjoyed reading them.

Having run the local activity coordinators network for over a year, I loved working with such creative people. The thought of extending this by working across the country appealed to me. I applied for the job and soon became part of the team. I couldn't believe it – this was my dream job. For years, I'd been telling anyone who would listen about meaningful activity, and now I was training activity coordinators. The daughter who had first found the reminiscence paper four years earlier and the training professional in me had come full circle.

I was thrilled to deliver training on various aspects of the activity coordinator role and, a little later, when I was asked to take on the role of Lead Trainer/Consultant, to develop other training content. The following year, other projects came along to support care homes that aspired to move away from those dreary activity programmes and my role developed further. Mum even got in on the action when I was asked if Daily Sparkle could use a couple of photos of her in one of their resources. *Who knew? A model at eighty-seven?*

The next few years were a joy. I was doing the work I loved, and I divided my time between various other projects and my work with Daily Sparkle. There was only a slight niggle. Every so often, a pang of guilt would emerge – I was successfully helping other organisations locally and nationally, but I still couldn't get things quite right for my own mum. *What sort of daughter am I?* I couldn't afford to dwell on those feelings – I focussed on the practical things I *could* do.

Back at Mum's home, I relaunched my mission to get people talking in the Lonely Lounge by using the *Daily Sparkle*. Whenever I went to visit her, my first task was to give out the reminiscence newspapers to the residents sitting in the lounge. The residents loved them and just having something to look at or chat about for a few minutes changed the energy in the room.

By now, I'd spent years on my quest to show carers that I wanted to help them. I tried it all: sing-alongs, Christmas carol services, Dementia Friends sessions, staff training and numerous projects with successive managers. In 2015 I found an accomplice in Rachel, whose grandmother and mother-in-law came to live in the home. Rachel was a kind and gentle woman, and she immediately took to The Lovely Rita. She joined me in many of my schemes, and particularly in the sing-along sessions where we belted out songs by The Carpenters. Mum would beam at me from her chair, and I'd remember what this was all about. Even after Rachel's relatives had passed away, she continued to be a regular visitor to the home. It comforted me knowing that Mum saw her smiling face every now and again.

Some schemes were more successful than others, but we celebrated every step forward. There always seemed to be something that stood in our way – be it staff absences or other priorities in the home. There was something else standing in my way too. I could never quite shake the feeling of being tolerated rather than welcomed.

I know now that that my feelings about Mum's care and my thoughts about how the home was run merged into one, and I foolishly tried to address both. I must have confused the care team. There was I, a family member, keen to get involved in a vastly different way to what they were used to. The different managers were always willing to let me launch my various schemes but perhaps they could have been more robust in supporting my efforts. What I didn't know – what I *never* knew – was how to be helpful without carers dismissing it as 'just Helen'. Once, when I made a comment about something or other, a staff member asked, 'are you saying that as a daughter or as a volunteer?' I didn't think that it mattered but their words showed me that it did.

Nevertheless, my split role had many benefits. I'd like to think that, primarily, I looked at care from Mum's perspective and as a relative who observed that care. My work now gave me a 360-degree view of how the wider care system worked and what residents should expect from care home life.

Chapter 25

From Pads to Podiatry:
What Worked, and What Didn't

2018

I had now been on the Experts by Experience journey for two years and was regularly taking part in inspections of care homes and other services. In 2018 I was asked to provide introductory and refresher training for other Experts carrying out that role. I loved training the next round of Experts and hearing the stories of what had brought them to the job. Many of them had joined the programme to improve an aspect of the care that, for them, hadn't been an entirely positive experience.

An unexpected bonus from working on this programme was my friendship with Debbie. Debbie had been an inspector of care services for several years before becoming an Expert by Experience in 2017. Her mum also lived in a care home so she, like me, had that 360-degree view of care from a personal and professional perspective.

Although her mum lived hundreds of miles away from mine, we swapped surprisingly similar stories about the puzzling situation we found ourselves in. We bonded over our shared frustrations and even created a name for the absurd care home world that we felt we occupied: 'Daughterville'. I know there are many sons, husbands, wives, partners and friends out there who support people who live in care homes, but for us, the name Daughterville summed up our situation. To us, Daughterville was a place where the rules of the outside world didn't seem to apply, where logic appeared to fall away, and our voices went unheard. Whenever we encountered another seemingly illogical event or ludicrous response from either of our parents' care homes, we shared the detail in our next phone call. That description makes the experience sound light and benign. It wasn't. Living in Daughterville was at best depressing, and at worst terrifying.

We endlessly questioned the real purpose of a care home. It had to mean more than keeping residents fed and medicated – with a few kind words now and again. What was the point in maintaining health if people were bored and lonely? We wanted care that helped our mothers to thrive NOT just survive.

What do you do when you know how the system *should* work but it doesn't? What do you do when you avail yourself of all the policies and procedures, yet get nowhere?

Debbie and I had countless conversations over the years, and I found in her someone who was also deep in the care home world trenches. She understood my dilemmas before I even voiced them. I recognised the anger straining her voice – because I felt it too. We almost finished each other's sentences because we knew how a particular story might end. She was my adopted sister in Daughterville.

I had already told her that my long-standing joke about writing a book called 'From Pads to Podiatry' was becoming a self-fulfilling prophecy and my life was dominated by monitoring either Mum's feet or her incontinence. We regularly debated about how the ways in which health and social care services were commissioned, managed and delivered had the potential to either help or hinder their patients' progress. In both our mums' experience it was a mixed bag.

From Pads …

Mum's continence pads only became one of my missions after she moved into a care home. Before that, everything was okay. I had long since resigned myself to the fact that the standard issue of products that came with her change in living arrangements weren't ideal. However, we supplemented these with the 'posh pads' that she paid for herself.

Five years later, when the ever-complex toilet arrangements in the home didn't work and we still found Mum frequently wet, I requested a continence review. She needed a prescription for better pads. I was warned by staff and fellow relatives that this process was not for the faint-hearted but, with limited options, I ploughed on.

The first hurdle was to negotiate the rules governing access to the continence service, which in our area differed between care homes and nursing homes. Before I entered Daughterville, I naively thought that all homes were the same and that it was simply different terminology – clearly, they weren't. Mum lived in a care home which meant that requests had to be made from the Senior to the continence service, but via the district nurse. Apparently, I wasn't allowed to contact them direct, so I waited for the protracted communication chain to run its course.

Once the request had been received, the first task was to assess Mum's fluid intake and output over a few days. Afterwards, I was informed that Mum needed to reduce her fluid intake as (according to the records) she consumed three and a half litres of liquid per day. 'What?' I said. 'Three and a half litres? That can't be right.' Alarm bells started ringing. The suggestion of limiting the fluid intake of a diabetic person – who was prone to UTIs – on the strength of information that I couldn't believe to be correct seemed crazy. I needed to check this out.

On my next visit to the home, I asked to check a fluid intake record. There in black and white was the perfect illustration of how, every day, Mum got a cup of tea at breakfast (250ml), then again at midday (same amount), a drink at lunchtime, then more tea mid-afternoon and so on. For the four days I looked at, it showed that she drank the same volume of liquid at the same time every day. Even with the home's fixed daily routines, this pattern seemed too perfect to me. I knew that I often found cold cups of tea left abandoned where Mum had presumably forgotten they were there. The records didn't reflect any missed intake at all. I told the Senior and (breaking the rules) contacted the continence team about my concerns. I hinted that, in case there had been any mix-up, perhaps we should address the issue of standard pads no longer meeting Mum's needs rather than *reducing her fluid intake to suit the pad allocation.*

We then embarked on what felt like a half-baked attempt at testing out different pads but, after months of miscommunication, the quest went cold. With other care issues to attend to, and the common-held belief that any success was improbable, I let it drop. The professionals didn't pursue it and neither did I.

The system was so complex and created so many barriers that – even with an unsatisfactory outcome – eventually I gave up. Even though Mum's needs justified better pads, I had learned the wisdom of the phrase 'choose your battles'. I spent what little funds Mum had on buying the pads that she needed, rather than going through the hassle of negotiating a fruitless process. It was a shameful example of a part of the care system which was so bureaucratic that patients or their relatives become worn down, to the point of giving up on a legitimate request.

Thankfully, some services worked better.

... to Podiatry

Mum's feet had always been a problem. Years of corns and ulcers along with aching, swollen feet and legs meant she needed special prescription shoes. She had poor circulation, and the skin on her legs was thin and sensitive. Suffice to say that she needed regular attention from the podiatry service.

After a few false starts in 2013, Mum came under the care of the outpatient diabetic centre at the local hospital where she had fortnightly appointments. Of course, Mum couldn't go alone, and I knew that the home couldn't release carers on such a regular basis. I decided that these visits were part of our outings, so every second week, Mum and I trooped off for her regular appointment – you could almost set your clock by us.

Not long after I'd had to give up with the pad scenario, I realised how important *this* service had become in keeping Mum well – both physically and emotionally.

Our visits usually followed the same pattern. I'd arrive at the care home, hoping that the Podiatry Gods had smiled upon me, and Mum would be ready. I'd swing into action to do the last-minute jobs: coat on, spritz of perfume, scarves and gloves and a quick flash of lipstick. Then it was into the car for the short drive to the hospital.

The way that everyone treated Mum was what made me grateful for this service.

We had attended the clinic so regularly that everyone knew the sweet, friendly old lady who had a smile for everyone. Usually, she was greeted with a 'Hello, Rita,' from the receptionist, and we'd take our seats in the waiting room.

Once we were called into the treatment room, the podiatrist made a fuss of Mum, telling her how smart she was, how nicely her hair was styled or how well she looked. Mum shrugged her shoulders at the compliments, but I could tell she was flattered. I beamed with pride and made a mental note to pass on the compliments to the carers.

As Mum lay on the treatment bed having corns, callouses and hard skin removed, she'd chatter away, amusing the podiatrist with her funny sayings. 'Tea clarty in the larty' was one of her favourites, but I still don't know what it meant. Sometimes I'd give her a magazine to distract her, and she'd read the words out loud in that polite sing-song voice. Despite any treatment that nipped at her feet, her twinkly smile filled the little room.

It was in those contented moments that I thought about what made this better than other services we had experienced. Firstly, I was grateful for their expertise. In the years that we had been going there, Mum's previously swollen feet and legs had reverted to normal size. Between her carers and the podiatrists, they had kept her diabetic feet in decent shape.

'These feet are probably the best I'll see today!' a podiatrist told me one morning. I beamed with pride and was quick to congratulate the Senior and carers when we got back to the care home.

However, it was their welcoming smiles, their interest in what Mum said and the compliments they paid her that all contributed to the visit going smoothly. My otherwise-jittery Mum knew that she was in a friendly place and felt included. I thought about the words that I'd learned years earlier. *It's not just what you do … it's how you make me feel.* That phrase stuck with me, and now, in both my personal and professional life, I have it in the forefront of my mind when observing any care.

In a care journey that often felt like a game of Snakes and Ladders – where at any point you could be elevated with joy or plunged into despair – this was a welcome relief. We probably visited the diabetic centre over two hundred times and, although it was a routine appointment, it was made better by the people who offered this service with empathy and respect. I was in no doubt that their compassionate approach helped both Mum and I sustain this important routine every two weeks for so many years and saved her from greater foot problems.

In this part of the 'Pads to Podiatry' tale, I saw the positive side to the health and social care system, which was empathetic and encouraging. Mum was respected and as a relative I was welcomed as a partner in care. That is how care should feel.

Chapter 26
Snakes and Ladders: All Change ... Again!
2018

The following year brought yet another change of management within Mum's care home. Carol, the previous manager, left and the deputy manager, Paul, grabbed the helm with both hands. This quietly spoken man, who had been promoted through the ranks, understood the complexities of each caring role and how the home operated. He also had first-hand experience of the highs and lows of working for the previous managers and seemed keen to make his mark. I was particularly impressed by how he was respectful to residents and relatives alike.

Over the course of a few years, the various Seniors I encountered fell into two categories: those who I felt I could rely on to get things done and others who seemed not to respect our concerns. Thankfully, all the Seniors who worked on Mum's floor, at this point, were very efficient in managing the day-to-day processes. Mum was always ready for her appointments and the important morning routine was in place most days. Kathy and most carers had a lovely relationship with Mum, whose quirky little ways they understood. I noticed that each one was particularly skilled in their own way.

• Dawn, who took the time to hold Mum's hand, look her in the eye and 'invite' Rita to join her for lunch – making her feel special.

- Grace, who had a bright and breezy way of tackling the toilet issues as an opportunity to 'freshen up' – reducing any embarrassment.

- Gill, who didn't gush but sat peacefully with Mum watching another snippet of Mamma Mia for the thousandth time – helping her stay calm.

- Kerry, who worked the night shifts. Her loving way towards Rita soothed my worries about whether Mum would be okay if she woke up scared in the middle of the night.

- Sarah, who was our original hairdressing star and had been promoted to a Senior. Throughout the years, she introduced Mum to her own children and grandchildren – making her feel loved.

I knew that, whatever else happened, Mum was held in extremely high regard there. It made me feel much more confident about her life in the home. It felt better.

We entered a period of relative stability. Yes, Mum was still deteriorating but she was happy and calm. At last, we had found a way to exist and made our peace with how care home life worked. I'd reluctantly accepted that activities in the home wouldn't now meet her needs but, when I was around, I made sure she had something to stimulate her. Equally, the carers knew to leave her music or a movie playing in the background, which seemed to soothe her. She still walked the corridors at times, but it was far less frequently or frantically.

My main concern, at that time, was around mealtimes. Mum's difficulties in bigger groups now extended to when she went into the dining room for her meals. As more of her skills failed, she seemed increasingly vulnerable there. She struggled to hold a knife and fork and sometimes used her fingers to eat. I worried about other residents making unkind comments – I'd seen that with other people years before.

There were often squabbles in the dining room – sometimes instigated by Mum, but often by others. I could see that having so many people at various stages of dementia in one area was a recipe for misunderstandings and upset. I asked if we could use the unused quiet lounge for small groups and was delighted when the manager said we could. I donated a dining table and, for a few months, it worked well. Mum loved the relative peace in that space and was free to eat away from judging eyes. At one point, the manager invited families to dine with their relatives and Ian and I took up the offer a few times – it felt lovely. One lady regularly had Sunday lunch with her mother in that room and often invited Rita too – I was grateful beyond words.

Unfortunately, as time went on, carers seemed keen to have everyone contained in one place, so residents were automatically ushered to the main dining room and the idea fell by the wayside. I despaired for Mum but, by now, knew how far I could go. We agreed that Mum could have her meals in her bedroom if she didn't feel happy in the dining room.

She was now very contented in that cosy room. We had recently brought her table from storage at my house, and when she wasn't having her meals there, she might be painting. When it was good, I was joyful, and felt that I could breathe. It still felt like a game of Snakes and Ladders but now there were far more ladders than snakes.

Every now and again there was a flashpoint around incontinence, the food, or other irritations but, generally, the atmosphere had improved. I knew the manager was slowly changing the culture of the home but that took time.

Some great events were happening in the home, and I was pleased that there was now a livelier atmosphere throughout. The downside was that these didn't often extend to Mum's floor, or they weren't aimed at those with more advanced dementia. The imbalance between the different floors had annoyed me for years and at Christmas time we saw a perfect example. The ground floor reception area was like a winter wonderland – festooned with all manner of decorations. However, the first floor decorations were so sparse that one of the carers brought some in themselves to cheer the place up. In solidarity, I donated some too, but not before pointing out the unfairness to the manager.

We focussed on the positive relationships and minimised other worries. When things went wrong, we concentrated on the benefits of Mum being looked after by people who cared *about her* – as well as *for her.* Whenever I was frustrated, I brought myself back to the reality of our options. Mum's home was a nice home that had received a 'Good' rating at their last inspection. Yes, we might find somewhere better at some aspects of care, but would they be worse at others? Would I be unsettling Mum only to replace one set of worries with a new one? I couldn't take that chance. By now, I had visited lots of care homes in my professional capacity and worked with numerous care teams, locally and nationally. I admired and respected their hard work and dedication but saw a familiar pattern in the way homes ran on a day-to-day basis. If we were ever to risk moving Mum, it would only be to somewhere that operated in a dramatically different way.

I started to feel hopeful and turned my attention to addressing my own needs. I knew I couldn't take care of Mum if I was unhealthy myself, so I embarked on another diet and eventually lost the weight I had piled on. I felt healthier and happier.

For a good two years we had relative calm and Mum was finally settled. It was each individual carer who made such an enormous difference and kept us committed to staying there – we thought she'd be there until the end.

In the game of Snakes and Ladders, we didn't realise there was trouble ahead.

*****

Staff retention in the care sector is notoriously poor and, although we enjoyed periods of stability, this home was no exception. Every now and again, there were a flurry of changes which derailed our progress. Carers who were once 'the new kids on the block' suddenly were the more experienced ones and the pecking order changed. Inexperienced carers or those unfamiliar with that floor did their best to carry out care tasks, but it caused delays and disruption. Things that had been embedded in Mum's care for years inexplicably stopped happening.

The relative calm we had enjoyed started to disappear and my worry returned as I noticed things changing. Mum's morning routine was missed for days on end, and she would look scraggy and have a temper to match. The Seniors reported, 'your mam isn't in a good mood today,' more frequently and I sensed things slipping backwards. Aileen could barely get through Mum's bedroom door without being shouted at. It seemed that everything we had worked hard to achieve over the previous six years was disintegrating.

I sensed another change looming once our gentle manager had been given extra duties – working at Head Office and across the company. This was great news for him, but I was uneasy about the knock-on effect on Mum's care. The Seniors were great but the situation with carers looked very fragile. Some left, some were promoted and others … well, I don't know what happened, but they weren't around. My worst fears were confirmed when it was announced that the manager would not be returning and was leaving the company altogether. *Not again!* I thought. I couldn't face another 'all change' moment and couldn't bear more instability for Mum. The Snakes and Ladders game had hit another snake.

The acting manager was very efficient in running the home, but I had misgivings about other things. I was in no mood to wrestle with another change in management style. Mum's care started to feel fragile again and I wondered if we could weather any further disruption. The answer to that question was to come in a few short months.

2019: The end of the road

One day in April, Aileen called me from the car park of Mum's home – she was livid. Unusually, for her, she had visited at teatime and was in Mum's room when she saw the meal that was offered.

'It was awful, Helen,' she said. 'Mam had the choice of soup or kippers. The soup was watery and there wasn't anything to go with it.'

'Bloody hell,' I said, 'just soup? Nothing else?'

'I know, and it was packet soup, Helen. It was so thin and watery that Mam didn't know what to do with it.'

'So, what did she eat eventually?'

'Well, in the end, I had to ask for some sandwiches to go with it.'

'But … what the hell would have happened if you weren't there?' I raged. 'She would have been starving if that's all she had 'til supper time. Mam wouldn't have been able to tell them that she was still hungry.'

Mum had a good appetite and I feared that our diabetic mother would be ill with only soup to sustain her. I was doubly furious as I'd written to the manager eighteen months previously to request that the food in the home be reviewed. I'd been put off repeatedly.

'That's it!' Aileen said. 'I'm complaining to the owner.'

The next day, she did exactly that and a meeting was arranged with the acting manager and a member of the head office senior team. As soon as the meeting started, I knew we were in trouble. Aileen was understandably in a defensive mood and insisted that the soup was from a packet. The manager claimed that it wasn't – the company didn't buy packet soup. Neither side budged. *We are wasting time on this!* I thought.

'Isn't the point that it was so thin and watery that it *looked* like packet soup? It doesn't matter if it was or wasn't – can we all agree that it wasn't the right quality?'

Before long we were in another circular debate about the absence of supplementary sandwiches. I couldn't stand it.

'Our point is,' I said, 'that Aileen had to specifically ask for them. Mam isn't able to do that so if Aileen wasn't there – she would have only had the soup. It wasn't enough food.'

The disjointed discussions went back and forth so much that my head spun. For every point we made they came back with banal statements, the importance of quality assurance, the competence of the kitchen staff, the chef's experience and so on … none of it addressing the specifics of the complaint. I sensed they hadn't truly grasped our point. The meeting was a jumble of platitudes and half apologies without any plans to stop it from happening again. Worse still, the meeting ended with a crushing afterthought delivered by the head office manager. She casually announced that Mum was

227

due a personal review soon and that she may need to move to the Dementia Unit upstairs. Aileen and I looked at each other in shock.

'What?' I said. 'This meeting isn't about Mum's review or which floor she lives on – it is a complaint about the food.'

The same gut-wrenching feeling returned. This felt like a veiled threat that Mum would be moved, and I saw the panic in Aileen's eyes. We cut the conversation short and left. We had come to the meeting in good faith and now left with more worries than when we started. Outside, in the car park, Aileen turned to me.

'She'll be going up there over my dead body,' she said.

'Mine too. It is NOT happening.'

Mum had lived here for six years, and whatever gripes we had, we didn't want her moved to the second floor. We didn't have anything against the staff up there, but we didn't think it was right for Mum. Although her dementia was progressing fast, I knew that she would still be better off where she was with staff she knew. If that was taken away, there was no hope.

The following days were sheer torture for us. It seemed that, by complaining, we had opened a can of worms that exposed Mum to all kinds of scrutiny. Arrangements that had been in place for years were picked over and questioned. It was so unsettling that I feared they were either gearing up to move Mum upstairs or kick her out altogether. We had imagined that Mum would see her days out in this home, surrounded by those who loved her and treated her well, but now everything was slipping away. After one particularly difficult day, I came to a conclusion that had been staring me in the face for years.

It was one of those 'your mam isn't in a good mood today' days and I couldn't settle her. I'd tried everything and was on the verge of tears for most of the visit. My head was filled with worries about the recent events, the latest care hiccups as well as Mum's ongoing deterioration. When it was time to go, as I walked towards the lift, I felt an overwhelming heaviness within me. For some unknown reason, I remembered the words the deputy manager had said, more than six years earlier, when we visited the home for the first time.

'We never want you to leave here with a heavy heart.'

The words stung. *How many times have I trudged out of here with just that – a heavy, heavy heart?* I thought, as I stepped inside the lift. I willed myself not to cry. *Just get through the hall and out the door.* I didn't want anyone to see me in tears. As I passed the office, I shouted a cheery 'bye', pressed the code into the door pad and heard the click that released me. I had made it. Once inside the car I drove to a nearby side street, turned off the engine, placed my head on the steering wheel and sobbed. I could not do this any more.

I was more than six years into this episode of our life and had tried everything to shake this horrible feeling I had about it. Nothing worked.

Once I'd cried it all out, I tried to think clearly. The question that I had wrestled with for more than six years was there again – s*hould we move her?* This time I considered it properly, not pushing it away. There were numerous explanations for why we stayed stuck in that unsatisfactory situation for so long. Even with all the mind-numbing frustrations, every year there was a reason to continue on the same path. Now it felt different.

That's when the realisation hit me. This home was never going to change so I had to. When I imagined the years ahead of us, with Mum's dementia worsening and the prospect of me having to fight for God knows how long – it filled me with dread. Aileen and I had already discussed the dire situation we were in. We had nothing to lose now – if they were hell-bent on disrupting her life at some stage, I wasn't going to wait around.

Unbeknown to Aileen, I decided I'd do some digging around an option that I'd thought was beyond us.

*****

I made a call to the manager of the purpose-built specialist dementia care home that I'd visited several times as part of my work. I remembered the time I first spoke about it with her when she was running another home. She'd told me about the plans to build it sometime in the future and I'd joked, 'I don't know if Mam will last that long!'

By the time it had opened, and I saw the natural effortless way of living there, I was envious but clung to the notion of 'better the devil you know'. I hadn't considered moving her – until now.

I explained our situation and the manager agreed that Mum could visit, and they would assess whether they could meet her needs. I arranged the first visit in July. It felt like an interview – for Mum and for me. I had never imagined that Mum would live anywhere else and now I was contemplating the unthinkable. I knew this type of care could help her, but would they take her? I didn't dare get our hopes up.

I told Aileen what I'd done, and she said she'd support whatever I thought best. She reasoned, 'well, if they're planning to move her at the other place, what does it matter if she goes somewhere completely new?' Sometimes Aileen simplified things much better than me. I checked with Barbara – she trusted our judgement and agreed that we couldn't go on as we were.

The day before our visit, I asked the carers to make sure that Mum had a nice outfit on as we were going to have a day out together. I didn't say where and felt guilty for deceiving them. On the day itself, I was so nervous and desperate for it to go well. Mum looked smart as usual, and I drove the short distance to the new home. The bright welcoming entrance was a delight and the smiling face on the receptionist immediately made Mum feel at ease. She didn't realise the significance of the visit – she was well beyond that stage – but simply responded to the warm atmosphere and the smiley faces in front of her.

We made our way through to one of the small households. There was a large, bright kitchen/dining area with residents happily sitting at a low-level breakfast counter. Opposite was a comfortable lounge area and I helped Mum take a seat on one of the sofas. As I parked her walking frame out of the way, I noticed that a member of staff had already cosied up beside Mum and was chatting to her. I saw that she had made direct eye contact with her and held her hand as they spoke. My lovely mother glowed with happiness at this gentle attention. I looked around me and there seemed to be lots of carers milling about – much more than at Mum's place. Across the room a visitor had arrived with his dog. As the gentleman and his wife talked to each other the dog lay contentedly at their feet.

Other residents and staff said hello to us and there was an air of calm. Residents who liked to walk freely could do so between each household as there were no locked doors and keypads to restrict them. I thought of the restrictions in Mum's home that caused more grief than any safety measure they imposed. This felt a much more natural way to live.

The arrangement was for me to leave Mum to have lunch there so that they could assess her. I left my contact number with the House Leader in charge of that household and made my way to the car. As I drove away, I had the sense that I'd forgotten something … it was so unusual for me to leave her anywhere. I busied myself at home for the next couple of hours but couldn't stop myself from thinking, *I hope she's okay.* Later I returned – to see a happy and sleepy Mum.

The next day I rang the manager and, after a couple more visits and discussions about fees, we got the call to say that Mum could move in. I was thrilled and couldn't wait to tell Aileen and Barbara. By then, Aileen had visited the home with Alan and couldn't believe how natural and homely it was.

A date was set for her to move in – it was going to happen – there was no going back. I now had to give notice at her current home.

*****

Telling the carers broke my heart. Out of courtesy, I went to the acting manager's office first, but she wasn't available, so the deputy came to see me. She had been one of the original kind carers who was always lovely to Mum. Seeing the worried look on my face, she probably thought that I was there to raise yet another issue.

'I've got something to tell you, Sarah ...' I gulped to take a breath; I knew this was going to be hard.

'What's wrong?' There was genuine concern in her voice.

'We've decided that it's time for Mam to move on.' I barely got the words out and the tears were rolling down my cheeks. She looked shocked. 'I know you'll miss her, but we've got to do the right thing for her.' The tears were in full flow now.

'Where's she going?' she said.

I explained about the new home and how they could offer her the level of staff attention and the type of care she needed as she declined. I didn't tell her that I felt sad to be taking my mum away from the remaining team who genuinely loved her, but our safety net had gone, and we knew more changes could occur at any time. We had done all we could over the previous six years to get the care Mum needed at each stage of her dementia. Now, with so much uncertainty here, I had to act.

I composed myself again and we hugged. I asked if I could personally tell the Seniors on the first floor – I felt I owed them an explanation. They knew I respected them, but they also knew that there were things I'd been unhappy about lately and that I was frustrated again.

As before, my voice cracked, and I cried as I told each one. Word spread around the building quickly and other carers asked why Mum was moving. I'm sure some were furious with me. They loved her – she'd lived there for six-and-a-half years, and I knew they'd miss her terribly. I explained as kindly as I could, but couldn't stop myself from thinking, *if you'd done the small things that I'd been asking – begging for, for years – then I wouldn't be doing this.*

It was breaking my heart to take The Lovely Rita away from them, but I knew that as her dementia got worse life would be harder for her. She would need more intensive support and I couldn't be certain I'd agree with their approach. If we'd stayed, my fight would have continued and it would have become a nightmare. Despite the pain I was causing, I had to do it. It was over – it was time to move on.

Part 3

A Renewed Hope, Covid and Beyond

Chapter 27
Home Sweet Home
2019

It was early September 2019 when, at the age of eighty-eight, Mum moved into her new care home. We had made the decision and were confident it was the right thing to do – but that didn't stop me from worrying over whether she'd survive the upheaval. Neither did it stop the overwhelming sadness I felt at the prospect of leaving the staff and other residents. I had grown to love each interesting character and they'd become part of my life. I couldn't bear the thought of never again bounding into the lounge to say good morning to them, or joking about my latest mishaps and adventures.

In the weeks leading up to moving day, I had been busy preparing the way for what I hoped would be a seamless transition. I was astounded at the sheer volume of possessions Mum had accumulated but, this time, I had no one else to blame but myself. I'd been the one buying every trinket, sparkly bag, magazine and whatever else I thought might stimulate her. I took the items that I thought she wouldn't miss during the last couple of weeks to my house. From there, Aileen and I decided on their fate – either joining Mum in her new life or off to be recycled. Of course, the old faithful recliner chair was safe but was having the deep clean of its life before I delivered it to her new pad.

The day before the big move, I transferred her treasures and, just as I had almost seven years earlier, decorated her new bedroom with pictures, photos, ornaments and flowers. It looked so inviting that, as I passed carers on the way out, I said, 'don't worry – if Rita doesn't want to live here – I will.'

The day of the move started badly, despite having agreed a plan with the care home manager to minimise any disruption for Mum. Aileen and Alan were due to pick her up midmorning, say their final goodbyes and take her for a coffee. That gave me time to meet the removal men (who were taking the bed and a few bulky items) and guide them between the two homes. Once at the new place, I'd make up the bed in the bright quilt cover that she'd recognise, before her arrival at lunchtime. My phone rang at around 10.30 am. It was Aileen.

'Helen, Mam's in a right state – she's refusing to get ready.'

'Shit! What's wrong?'

'She's full of hell and telling everyone to bugger off.' Aileen described all the tactics they'd tried to ease her out of her bad mood – to no avail.

'God, that's all we need,' I said. 'Right, how about I come up and see if a change of face might help?'

I grabbed my coat and arrived at the home fifteen minutes later. As soon as I walked in the room, I spotted what was likely to be the source of Mum's agitation. In their haste (or, if I'm being kind, efficiency) to pack for her departure, a member of staff had stripped her bed and piled all her remaining belongings on top of it. I winced at the undignified heap of plastic bags, astounded that anyone wouldn't realise how it could affect Mum. *Leaving her sitting in this mess wasn't part of the plan*, I thought. *No wonder she is out of sorts.* She was probably baffled as to what the hell was going on around her. Here was a lesson in how to further disorientate an already confused lady with dementia.

Stunned into silence, I looked at Aileen. I could see that, like me, she was struggling to contain her fury, but we didn't dare let Mum catch our mood. We had to concentrate on calming things down. After several attempts to sweet-talk her into getting ready we had to accept that it wasn't going to happen yet, and now it was almost lunchtime.

'How about we leave Mam to have something to eat and have a nap,' I said, 'then we'll try again later?'

'Good plan.' Aileen agreed to come back later. Meanwhile I notified the new home of our delay.

Our tactic worked. Mum woke up a few hours later, a totally different woman – all sweetness and light. She greeted Aileen with a smiley 'hello pet' and was perfectly happy to get dressed and leave. Aileen told me later that their departure was low key as she was still furious with those who had 'despatched' a resident so thoughtlessly. She was in no mood to have polite conversations, so headed out the door without fuss. I understood her anger but was saddened that, after almost seven years of living in this home, Mum had left without much acknowledgement. I'm not even sure whether anyone had the chance to say goodbye.

Her welcome at the new home couldn't have been more of a contrast as staff beamed at her when she arrived. We sat at the breakfast bar in the kitchen area and chatted with other residents and carers. Mum still loved to walk, so later we explored our way around the broad airy corridors, without the constraints of locked doors and keypads. Here, she could walk freely from household to household, marvelling at the lovely things she spotted. We found comfortable corners to sit quietly where soft toys and other items had been cleverly placed to stimulate a passing resident. We did a few circuits before returning to lounge.

After teatime, we went to Mum's room, and I showed her all her treasures in their new location. Her soft smile of contentment reassured me that we had done the right thing. I hoped that feeling would last. By early evening, the events of her busy day took their toll – she shut her eyes and was out for the count.

When I visited the next day, Mum was bright and breezy and, as the following days and weeks passed, she adjusted to her new life. The entire building felt different and much more homely. Here, it felt like everyone was living together in a more connected way than in the other home. *This is what I want for her,* I thought, as I absorbed the atmosphere they had created. I saw carers relaxing and spending time with residents in a natural and easy way. The higher staff ratios meant that carers had time to spend with individuals which created a warm and calm feeling. All the necessary care tasks still got done but they seemed to happen in the background as part of carers and residents happily mingling together.

It was the responsibility of all staff to provide stimulating and meaningful activity for residents, so there were no gripes as to whose job it was. The carers seemed fully on board with this concept, and I saw that in various parts of the home there was usually something happening. They seemed to understand the importance of those low-key activities with one or two residents which seemed gentle and natural. Residents were free to potter in any part of the home without being asked 'Where are you going?' It felt less controlling and I'm sure the residents must have sensed that.

Mum now spent more of her time in the lounge or kitchen area with others, rather than holed up in her bedroom as had been the way in her previous care home. After a few weeks of getting used to the comings and goings around her, she relaxed. The calm and peaceful atmosphere soothed her and the tension that I'd felt, whenever she was in the lounge in the other home, was gone.

We settled into a new routine. Mum made friends with other residents and found companions to sit with in various areas. We were optimistic for the future, and I especially looked forward to the following summer. Her bedroom had French doors which opened onto a small patio area, leading to a huge secure garden around the perimeter of the home. This allowed Mum to walk with the freedom I'd wanted for her for years. Aileen and I talked of buying a couple of chairs for the patio and I imagined us sitting together in the sunshine. My hopes soared for this next part of her journey. We had done it. She had survived the move and we would make this next phase work.

We were so confident in Mum's new life that when Christmas rolled around, we changed arrangements that had been in place for years. Aileen and I usually took turns at hosting the Christmas Day celebrations and, of course, Mum was always with us for the full day. Recently, we had seen her struggle with car journeys and using the stairs in either of our homes was now out of the question. With a tinge of sadness – but comforted in the knowledge that she would be pampered all day – we decided that it was best if she stayed at what had quickly become *her home*. On Christmas morning, we visited with gifts, and I felt relieved that I had finally reached a point where I could walk away from her without that heavy heart.

*****

The start of 2020 was busy. I was piloting a new training course and working away from home a lot. I also had a holiday booked. It was only ten days in Tenerife with Ian, but I looked forward to being in the sun. I arrived back from two days working in Ireland with one day to spare in which I had to take Mum to a podiatry appointment.

On February 20th 2020, I took Mum to the clinic, as usual, but this time in a wheelchair taxi. She could still walk with her frame, but the problems with getting in and out of the car made using her wheelchair for appointments a no-brainer. She could be wheeled straight from her room, into the taxi, into the clinic and returned home without any hassle. I sat in the back of the cab that morning, holding her hand and rubbing her small bony fingers inside the bright red gloves that I'd bought for her. She was wrapped up in her navy padded coat with so many layers underneath that she looked like the Michelin Man. I gabbled on, in what had now become one of our one-sided conversations. I'd noticed, since Christmas, a further deterioration in her speech as her sentences got shorter and more jumbled.

The appointment went well. A lovely podiatrist tended to Mum's feet and, as usual, we felt welcome. There were no problems with her toes, so we were quickly back in the taxi and returned home in time for lunch. I was relieved that there were no delays as I was a little preoccupied – I needed to get back home to finish off some outstanding work and get the last of my packing done. I kissed her, as I had done at least a thousand times before saying, 'See you in a couple of weeks, Mam.' I knew she was well cared for, so didn't have any misgivings about going away. I sent Aileen a text: *Our mamma is contented today. The carers got her ready and she looks lovely. Podiatrist says feet in good shape. All good with our world.*

Aileen would visit as usual, and I was confident that Mum would not be lonely in any way. *It's only for ten days*, I thought to myself as I drove away.

*****

The holiday in Tenerife was memorable. On day two, the island was hit by high winds and strong clouds of dust (apparently from Africa) which left a terracotta film across everything in sight. The pool area was damaged, and sunloungers lay haphazardly on top of each other. Within two days, the efficient resort staff returned everything to normal and you wouldn't know that there had ever been a storm.

On day five, Ian received a text message from one of his colleagues.

You're not in the hotel with the guest who has Coronavirus, are you?

'What's that?' I said. I'd been so busy that I hadn't paid much attention to any news before I'd left the UK, let alone an unknown virus. We switched on the TV and tuned in to Sky News to hear that the H10 Adeje Palace was on lockdown as the first case of the virus was confirmed in mainland Spain.

We'd passed a hotel in the same chain the day before but realised that the one in the report was a twenty-minute drive away from us – we were fine. We metaphorically shrugged our shoulders and continued the holiday in blissful ignorance. A local shopkeeper said it was probably a big fuss about nothing – nothing to worry about here. I took that at face value.

Each day, we grew a bit more curious, as more cases emerged in the same hotel and then in other places around the world. You would think we would be scared by this … we weren't. It all seemed so far away. The world was different then; we all thought differently then. After our ten days were up, we boarded our flight and returned to the UK.

The next day, I innocently turned up to visit Mum, as planned. Thankfully, before I even entered the building, the manager, who was in the reception area, headed me off. Once she had established that I'd been to Tenerife she politely asked if I could delay my visit for fourteen days – just as a precaution. I was disappointed and, if I'm honest, thought it may be an overreaction. The outbreak had been in a hotel twenty minutes away from where I was, so it was unlikely that I'd be a risk. Of course, this was at the beginning of

March and none of us knew what was to come or how it would change our thinking forever. Despite my doubts, I was happy to do as she asked and patiently waited until I was allowed to visit on the 17th of March. That visit never took place as, on the 13th of March, the home was declared closed. Indefinitely.

This was the first time I hadn't seen my mum for more than a two-week gap in ten years. It was unthinkable. How would she cope? How would I?

Chapter 28
382 Days
2020

On the 16th of March 2020 the first government announcement was made. The Prime Minister, Boris Johnson, told us that we had to stop non-essential contact and travel. At the same time, care homes were ordered to close their doors to all visitors. I was shocked at the news but thought everything would be resolved fairly quickly. I resigned myself to the fact that I couldn't see Mum any time soon, so thought about the practical steps I could take to help her. I delivered toiletries and gifts for her and left them outside the reception door.

By the 23rd of March, we were told to 'stay at home' which, for me, notched up the fear a bit more. *Is this really happening?* Half the time I felt like I was in a scary movie. I knew Mum would have no knowledge of what was happening in the world – she was far beyond that stage and, for once, I was grateful for her dementia. I was comforted that she was safely tucked away and looked after. If she'd been living independently, I would have worried non-stop.

Aileen had underlying health conditions that meant she was at greater risk from coronavirus and had to follow the shielding rules. She was advised to stay at home and avoid all face-to-face contact for a period of at least twelve weeks. It frustrated her, but she had to comply. Each week, one of us spoke to the House Leaders on the phone to check how Mum was doing, and reported back to the others. We received regular email updates, and I was devastated when one confirmed that there was a Covid outbreak in the home and residents were confined to their own rooms. I rang the manager straight away, who reassured me that staff would be checking Mum frequently – yet I still worried about how this extra isolation would affect her.

With nothing else to do and nowhere else to go, we stayed home. Ian and I took comfort in our permitted daily walks and, like the rest of the country, dabbled in some minor DIY projects. Each week I delivered an A4 postcard to Mum that I'd created by printing out a postcard template on one side and a photo on the front. I sent her messages telling her what we were doing, that we loved her and couldn't wait to see her. We waited it out.

On one sunny April morning, I was painting the garden shed when the House Leader from Mum's household rang. She explained that Mum had a high temperature, a cough and was struggling with her breathing. She thought that it might be Covid but was waiting for the paramedics and would notify me when they arrived.

Stunned, I hung up the phone, thinking, *I can't believe we will lose her this way*. I phoned Aileen and Barbara to share what little information I had and reassured them that I would call back as soon as I had more news.

When the phone rang again, it was one of the paramedics who had checked Mum over. Her oxygen levels were very low, but they couldn't say whether it was Covid or not. They asked if I wanted her to be taken to hospital. I didn't know. I knew that in ordinary times we never wanted our confused mum going to hospital, but these weren't ordinary times. *Would a hospital in the middle of a pandemic be safe for her? Realistically, could she be looked after at the home?* I had to answer. I instinctively knew what my sisters would want so agreed that, if she could be given help for her breathing, she should stay at the care home. I hung up, hoping that I'd made the right choice.

Within minutes, the phone rang again. This time it was one of the senior team at the home. They explained that, if Mum did have Covid, I could visit her, wearing full Personal Protective Equipment (PPE). Before a decision could be made, they needed to check with the out-of-hours GP, and then get back in touch. *This is serious – they must think she'll die.* I waited again, all the while agonising over how I could visit her safely without bringing anything back home to my asthmatic husband. *I'll have to do it*, I thought, *I've got to see her.*

In the early evening, the House Leader rang back. She had strange news. 'I've just been into your mam's room to check on her symptoms, ready to give them to the out-of-hours doctor,' she said.

'Yes …?' I dreaded what was coming next.

'Helen, she is fine. She hasn't got one symptom – not one. She's a bit tired but that's it!'

'Oh, thank God!' I said, the weight of the last few hours finally eased. 'What do you think it was?'

She was as puzzled as I was and didn't know why it had happened. We agreed to wait to see how Mum was the following morning and I updated my sisters.

The next day, I phoned the home and a carer confirmed that she was fine. She was out of bed and eating her breakfast as normal. It appeared that our wonderful mother hadn't had a potentially life-threatening brush with Covid after all. I laughed at Mum's unceasing resilience … even in the face of a deadly virus. Perhaps, if Covid *had* come calling, she had told it to 'bugger off' as well.

I was relieved that had she not succumbed to the worst that we could imagine but, as the weeks of separation turned into months, the House Leaders informed me of her continued deterioration. At first, I heard that she could no longer feed herself. Within weeks, they informed me that Mum couldn't walk or even support her own weight when standing – she now needed a hoist to move her. This was a worrying decline and I wondered what was next.

After the recent scare and a tearful call to the care home manager, she suggested I could see Mum through the garden gates for five minutes. This was well before care home visits were even on the horizon, so I was grateful for the gesture. That afternoon, as the carers wheeled Mum towards me, I called out her name. The bright shawl around her shoulders and blanket across her knees made her look like a fluffy little bundle. Her mop of hair was styled, and she was wearing a little make-up.

'Look Rita, there's your Helen,' one of the carers said excitedly, pointing in my direction. Although Mum was looking at me, something about her seemed different. She seemed vacant and puzzled as to what was going on. When I spoke, she didn't seem to notice who was talking and instead turned to the carer standing next to her. Physically, she looked very well, but even in the brief time I was there I could tell there had been a mental deterioration since I'd last seen her in the February. After the promised five minutes, I said goodbye. I was worried but thankful to have seen her at all.

A couple of weeks later, I was allowed back for another snatched five-minute gate visit, and Aileen – who was also struggling with not seeing Mum – came along too. She was still following the latest shielding rules, so we took turns at standing near the gate – keeping to the required two metres apart from each other and Mum. It was another kindly gesture, but afterwards we were told that we would now have to wait until a proper visiting regime was in place.

In June, with no other options open to us, I arranged to call Mum using Skype. After a couple of false starts the connection picked up and I saw one of the carers sitting close to Mum.

'Look, there's your Helen,' she said.

Mum smiled and stared directly into the screen. I was surprised that she knew where to look.

'Hello Mam,' I said. 'You look beautiful.' She did. Once again, her hair was nicely curled, and this time she was wearing a brightly coloured top. She wore one of her many beaded necklaces and matching earrings. Not only did she look the very picture of health, but she also seemed more alert than when I'd seen her briefly at the gate. I was relieved.

'It's Helen here!' I said. 'It's so lovely to see you, Mam!'

She mouthed a few words, but I couldn't make out what she was saying.

'Do you want to say hello to your Helen?' the carer said.

'Helen,' Mum said softly.

'Yes! Mam, it's your Helen,' I almost shouted at the screen. 'How are you doing? You look so well.'

Her gentle smile spread across her face as she looked up towards the carer who was already telling me that Mum was indeed doing well. *What a relief.*

'Isn't it great that we can see each other?'

I babbled on, fully aware that this was going to be a one-sided conversation. I knew not to ask her about what she'd been doing or any other specific details. Instead, I told her about what I'd been doing at home, exaggerating every point to make it sound far more exciting than my own locked-down life was.

The Skype call only lasted ten minutes but, after it was over, I was floating on cloud nine. I had seen her, and she looked well. She had gazed at the carer so lovingly that I could tell that she felt safe in her care. Despite the worries – I was comforted by knowing that she was being cared for by kind people in a cosy, calm environment. Individual staff in the other home had been lovely, but here I knew that everything was better organised to cater for her as her dementia progressed. I hung up, thinking: *At last, she feels at home somewhere - she really belongs there.* She looked relaxed so now *I* could relax.

Later that month, I received the much-awaited email from management saying that garden visits would start the following week. We would be allowed one thirty-minute visit per week but would have to wear face masks and gloves and stay a metre away from Mum. We weren't allowed to hug her or even touch her hand. Despite this, I was thrilled at the prospect of seeing her properly and, as soon as the booking system opened, I secured a slot for Ian and me on the first day.

On the day of the visit, I was both excited and nervous. A carer escorted us through the garden to the two chairs positioned at the required distance from where Mum's wheelchair would be placed. Minutes later, the House Leader brought her out. As he parked the wheelchair, I noticed that she was stooped forward – her head facing downwards. I knew she wouldn't be able to see me like that. Taking care not to get closer than allowed, I slid off the garden chair and sat cross-legged on the path directly in her eye line. As before, she was smiling and looking well-groomed, but she looked different again. She wasn't wearing her false teeth and their absence made the bottom of her face sink inwards. Her words were disjointed half-words and she didn't respond to anything I was saying. Still, I was so happy to see her that I nattered enough for both of us.

The garden visits became our lifeline but weren't ideal. Of course, I was grateful for any chance to see her but, for someone with Mum's advancing dementia, they were a disappointing substitute for close contact in familiar surroundings. A gazebo that had (with good intentions) been erected to provide shelter was, in reality, ineffective. The canvas flapped around and offered little protection from the northeast winds that blew, even on a sunny day. Worse still, the flapping distracted Mum and added to her confusion. She must have found it odd, to be taken out of the comfortable lounge to sit outside in front of two strange beings wearing face masks. Despite this, I loved seeing her in person and knew how important it was to keep these visits up. I pushed away unwelcome thoughts that, as we couldn't get near to her, Mum might not be benefitting from the visits as much as we'd hoped. At a time when all our lives were curtailed, we had to make the best of what was on offer. I prayed that, at some level, she sensed that her family were there.

Away from the care home, and when restrictions allowed, I walked on the beach with my friend, Julie, and her dog, Ada. Julie's dad had gone into a care home the previous year and she was equally frustrated. We shared our lockdown woes, swapping stories about the latest events and complaining about the inconsistencies in how homes approached the rules. Homes, situated less than five miles apart, had vastly different rules that created a postcode lottery as to whether you were allowed to see your loved one or not. It made me fume – yet again.

Julie understood because she'd now joined Daughterville. During one of our walks, she told me that it wasn't until her dad went to live in a home that she realised what I'd meant when I'd moaned about care home life for the previous seven years. While she'd sympathised at the time, she now understood the frustration experienced when a loved one lives within the care system. It turns even the most forthright of us into submissive wrecks, and during the Covid pandemic even more so.

To give Mum's home their due, they were doing what they thought best and provided opportunities that I knew other care homes in the area were not. In the late summer, I think even the care home management could see how ineffective the gazebo was and allowed us to meet in a large airy annex area adjoined to the main building. Aileen's period of shielding was now over, so she was also allowed to visit but, with one visit allowed per resident per week, we had to take turns. The indoor visits were better at protecting Mum from the cold but the strict thirty-minute distanced meeting did nothing to stop her rapid deterioration. Our mother had been used to almost-daily family visits for the previous seven years and, in my opinion, the long-term separation was accelerating her decline. I'd spent years advocating stimulation and occupation to benefit those with dementia and knew how its withdrawal was damaging. It was five months since I'd even touched Mum's hand, and each time I saw her, I noticed a change in her physical and mental state. I now questioned the wisdom of continuing with a national policy of 'protect from Covid' at all costs but, like millions of us, had no choice but to follow the rules.

Christmas 2020 came and went with no visits allowed at all. This was another first. I prayed that she was beyond sensing our absence on the day itself but felt that the rules were inhumane.

By January 2021, with Covid vaccines being rolled out, Mum's home provided an indoor visiting booth and extended the visits to one hour. The temporary structure was positioned inside the main area of the home, but it could be accessed from the outside doors. This meant that we could visit indoors safely, albeit with Mum sat on one side of a Perspex window, and us on the other.

Despite my initial enthusiasm, the reality of the booth visits was that they offered little opportunity for connection between me and Mum. I'd arrive full of enthusiasm, with Ian and our collection of items to stimulate her during the visit. Bright flowers, large photos, and music on my phone – we tried anything to get a reaction from her. A carer would wheel Mum to her side of the Perspex window, and I'd spend the next hour trying to catch her eye – even for a second. My darling mum rarely looked up, didn't smile or even notice that I was there. Most of the time, her head was down and her eyes were closed. I knew that her advanced dementia now meant that she was in a far-removed place mentally. It was likely that she was unaware of much beyond her peripheral vision that would be extremely limited now. I was fighting a losing battle. To make a connection with her now, I needed to get close to her, look into her eyes and hold her hand. This still wasn't a meaningful visit for Mum.

Part of me felt guilty for wanting more, when I knew that thousands of relatives weren't even getting this far with visits. The other part raged at the ineffectiveness of what we had. I appreciated each step the home had taken but the reality was that I'd spent almost a year simply 'viewing' my mother.

*****

I was infuriated by the delays and knew that, for my eighty-nine-year-old mum, waiting this out indefinitely wasn't an option. I did what little I could to call for change both locally and nationally. I wasn't against my mum's care home itself but was frustrated that, after so long, the rules hadn't changed to reflect the now fully vaccinated status of the residents. At the beginning of the pandemic, I had agreed with home lockdowns but, after seeing what a year of separation had done to Mum and others, felt we needed a different approach.

I had read about the thousands of people in care homes who were living without a connection to those they held dear. It was inconceivable that, after so long, we were still being kept apart. Whenever relatives challenged this approach, the stock response was 'we're protecting the residents', but after so long the solution was doing more harm than good. Care home teams did an excellent job and kept people safe, but they couldn't offer the same love that comes from a lifetime of knowing the person. People were living (and in many cases dying) without their loved ones by their side. It was horrendous. I wanted to scream 'sod the rules, sod protecting people from Covid – being apart from us is finishing her off anyway. She needs us NOW.' Some homes doggedly interpreted the rules without also applying logic, others felt their hands were tied and struggled to know what to do for the best. I understood the dilemma they faced and that everyone was making sacrifices, but I knew time was running out for our relatives.

As usual, I made comparisons to try to explain how it felt. I said to a close friend, 'Imagine if a mother sent their child – a vulnerable human – to school one day, and then got a phone call to say that they were keeping them there indefinitely (for their own safety). Imagine not being able to see your child for months, touch them or even reassure them if they are confused or scared. This is no different – just because the vulnerable person is in the latter stage of their life.' To further my point, I added, 'If it were children who were locked away – society wouldn't be politely waiting for the government to issue rules that allowed us to see them. Parents all over the land would be tearing down school buildings, brick by brick, to get to those they love. That's the urge I have – but I must wait.'

I became so angry that I went on local and national radio programmes to join the growing call for better visiting arrangements. I told one host, 'I don't want to have to wait until my mother is taking her dying breaths to tell her that I love her. I want to be with her and tell her that now.' I wanted to be with her before she lost what little cognitive function she had left. I supported national campaigns and attended meetings via Zoom to give an account of our own experience. I wanted everyone to know about the massive physical and cognitive decline that I felt that my mum had suffered because of the extended separation from her family. I was convinced that this had accelerated her dementia and I know hundreds of families had comparable stories. Even those who had gone into homes in relatively good health had fared badly in lockdown.

It seemed that those in power did not help. I felt that the government failed to fully appreciate the longer-term impact of their draconian rules on our loved ones. Yes, Mum had been protected from Covid, but her speedy decline was the price she paid. Even when newspapers were awash with horrifying stories of rapid deterioration in residents' health, they didn't seem to act quickly to change the rules. When updated guidance was eventually issued, adherence wasn't mandatory, so care homes made their own decisions. Thousands of heartbroken relatives and friends found themselves in a care home visit lottery. There was no logic to it.

At its heart, it felt like a violation of Mum's human rights, and I knew that if she hadn't been living in a care home I would have done things differently. If I'd had the option of managing the risk to my mum's life but, at the same time, wrapping her in the family love that she thrived on, I would have done it. I know that would have been my mum's choice too. *What is the point of living, if being apart from those you love is killing you slowly anyway?* After the vaccine roll-out, my choice would have been to dispense with the masks and the distance and hold her hand. As it was, every part of our connection to The Lovely Rita slipped away, as I watched her from behind a Perspex screen.

*****

Thankfully, Mum's care home continued to make progress. In March 2021, the addition of a purpose-built visiting room inside the main building opened up the long-awaited possibility of being able to hold Mum's hand once again. We still needed to book a visiting slot and wear full PPE, but it gave us the chance to communicate properly with her.

On Monday 8th March 2021, I waited nervously in that cosy little room with another bag of goodies for her. As Mum was wheeled in, I jumped up to greet her.

'Hi Mam,' I said.

'Hello,' she replied, her voice clear and strong. I reeled at the sound of her voice – it was so long since I'd heard her speak. She had never greeted me once during the other visits and, on most, hadn't uttered a word. I was sure that sensing someone close to her (rather than beyond a screen) made a difference. I was already overjoyed, and she'd been in the room less than thirty seconds.

I sat back on the chair but reached over to hold both of her hands. I hadn't touched her in 382 days. I knew the exact number because I had counted each day that we were apart. Although I had to wear latex gloves, I rubbed her tiny bony fingers as she locked her hands in mine. Just feeling her delicate little hands was a joy.

'Hello, my beautiful Mam,' I said. 'I love you so very much and I've missed you. It's lovely to be sitting with you. Isn't this a gorgeous room?' All that I'd learnt about communicating with people with dementia went out of the window as I babbled away.

Eventually, I settled down and looked at her properly. Unlike on the other visits, her eyes were open, so I was able to look directly into those warm blue eyes as I spoke to her. They no longer had that same twinkle to them, but nevertheless she smiled gently. In contrast, I had a huge grin on my face behind the paper mask and I hoped she could sense the happiness.

I showed her the bright yellow daffodils I'd brought for her.

'Look at these pretty flowers, Mam,' I said, and did a double-take when she nodded in response. *A reaction – this is great!*

A little later, I fished in my bag of goodies for something else. I'd recently been in touch with Kathy from the old care home and she'd emailed some photos of her baby which I'd printed out on A4 paper.

'Mam – I've got a photo of Kathy's baby. Look at this lovely little boy.' I placed the photo on her knee, and she grasped it with one hand and stroked the image with the other. *Another reaction.* I knew she wouldn't understand who was in the photo, but the colourful image made an impact. Whenever I'd held anything up to the Perspex window of the visiting booth, it went completely unnoticed. The difference in her reactions brought a tear to my eye.

Mum loved music, so later I played some Nat King Cole songs on my phone. She smiled as she heard the familiar tune, gently closed her eyes and they stayed closed for the rest of the visit – well, almost. At one point, she opened just one eye and stared directly at me. *There she is – my jokey Mam!* I laughed out loud. In fact, a bit too loud which made her open both eyes briefly, before shutting them again. It reminded me of how she always pulled faces and joked around – everyone loved her sense of humour. Even with her eyes closed, she clung firmly to my hands, occasionally picking at the latex of my gloves.

To the outside world, those tiny reactions would be insignificant, but to me there was a stark difference in the way Mum responded in this visit and the way it felt. Sitting close to her in that room gave me the opportunity to communicate with her in the ways that meant something to her now. Touching her hand, looking into her eyes, and using the music and bright coloured objects, helped me connect with her. I was elated and imagined that we would continue with these types of visits until I achieved my ultimate goal – to sit with her in her own bedroom. I didn't realise that my wish would be granted sooner than I thought.

Chapter 29

In Her Room

April 2021

A couple of weeks after that glorious day in the visiting room, the manager of the home rang to inform me of some changes that were about to take place. Mum was moving from her current household to another that was more suited to her needs. Her deterioration meant that she needed a higher level of support, and the other household could provide that sort of care. I was worried because I'd seen how comfortable Mum was with the carers who had looked after her since she moved into the home. At this stage of her dementia, I knew that, more than ever, she needed consistency, and the idea of any changes worried me. My reservations were allayed when the manager told me that a few staff were moving into this household along with Mum so there was some continuity.

She also announced that Mum could have one of us nominated as her Essential Care Giver to visit in her own bedroom two or three times a week. This new role had recently been introduced nationally as part of the government's Covid guidance. Aileen generously allowed me to be the nominated person and I was grateful for the gesture. This meant an end to scrambling to be one of the first to get through on the phone each week when the limited number of visiting slots were released. I could visit at a time when Mum was most likely to be alert and stay a little longer, without worrying that my allocated time would run out before she had even opened her eyes. Aileen could take my place for a weekly slot in the visiting room, and she would get to hold Mum's hand too. We were gradually getting nearer to normal visits for both of us – this was looking promising.

It was another significant milestone and that first visit in her bedroom was wonderful purely because of its intimacy. After over a year of uncomfortable, impractical arrangements, I was able to sit beside her, in her own space, while her favourite music played, and hold her hand. We sat cosily together with me offering a few words every now and again. This time no clock-watching.

Mum still slept (or had her eyes shut) for most of the visits but, on one occasion, I realised that if I gave her some of the chocolate buttons I'd brought, she'd open her eyes for a few moments. Even so, she seemed to look into space – as if she couldn't see me right in front of her. Her condition had worsened, and she looked only semi-conscious. On another day, I helped her take a drink of juice and to see her enthusiastically gulp each mouthful made my heart sing. I was like a new mother celebrating their child's every movement. For over a year, I hadn't seen her do anything other than sit in a chair, so I was encouraged by every little thing. I was determined that we were on the road to getting more time together and giving her more stimulation. I had plans.

The care staff were wonderful, and it comforted me when they told me of things she did when we weren't there. Mum wasn't capable of any major feats now but hearing even the smallest anecdote helped. A carer told me that, the night before my visit, she was tucking Mum up in bed and said, 'Rita, your daughter is visiting tomorrow,' and Mum had given her the biggest of smiles. I was thrilled that, at some level, she had responded to the word 'daughter'.

There were days when she slept for the whole visit and didn't open her eyes once. I was disappointed but, after the year we'd had, I treasured every moment in her bedroom. I was determined to get Aileen to experience the same, but we had to wait until the national guidance and the care home would allow it. I was working on it when an unexpected call changed everything.

A couple of weeks after the first bedroom visit, I was in Marks and Spencer, when my phone rang. It was Sandy, one of the managers from the home, trying to tell me something about Mum's circulation and that a wound on her foot wasn't getting any better. The store was noisy and wearing a facemask seemed to affect my hearing anyway.

'Sorry, I can't quite hear you,' I said.

She repeated the information, but everything still sounded a little disjointed. Somehow, amid the confusion, it suddenly dawned on me what she might be trying to tell me.

'Sandy – is this the thing that sometimes means that diabetics need to have an amputation? Is that what we're talking about?'

'Well, yes … sort of. We want you to be aware that the foot is not looking good, but we can have a chat early next week.'

'Oh, I see. Erm … thanks for letting me know. I'll talk to my sisters about it.'

I was in a daze, and hadn't fully taken the information on board, but called Aileen and suggested we contact Barbara. I then doubted what I'd heard and worried that I'd misunderstood.

'Aileen …' I hesitated. 'I'm not sure whether I've heard this properly. I don't know what we can tell Barbara at this stage. Let me talk to Sandy on Monday, to check I've got this right and then we'll call her.'

I visited Mum, as planned, the next day (Saturday), and took a quick peek at her foot. She was wearing trousers and tights so I couldn't see anything unusual. Again, I doubted my understanding of the situation. *Is it really worse? Perhaps I've got this wrong*, I thought. I had so many questions in my head. I texted Aileen: *If it's about her circulation – how do you improve the circulation for a person who is immobile?* I was confused as to what would happen next.

Aileen fretted that the home might not be able to manage Mum's ongoing decline and wondered if the Friday call was a precursor to them wanting to move her to a home with nursing facilities. I was sure that wouldn't be the case. For the last ten months, Mum had been hoisted and helped with her feeding – I couldn't see what would be different now, even if she did lose her foot.

On Monday, before I even had a chance to contact Sandy, Mum's GP called and explained everything. Mum's foot had lost all its circulation and essentially the limb was dead. Our options were either to have her admitted to hospital, or she could stay at the care home. If she went to hospital, it was unclear as to how they could treat her foot. It was unlikely that they would amputate, as there was no reasonable chance of rehabilitation and an operation of that sort on an eighty-nine-year-old was not a great option. However, if untreated, the poor circulation in the foot would eventually kill her. I asked the inevitable question. 'How long are we talking?'

'Your mum has probably got weeks or months to live, rather than years,' she said.

'Okay – I think I know what Mam would prefer but I'll speak to my sisters.'

A quick ring around confirmed the plan. We'd agreed years before that our confused Mum didn't fare well in hospital and now, in Covid times, we wouldn't even be allowed to visit. At least, at the home, they knew her and she was loved. They would take care of her until the end came and we could visit her regularly.

The next day, I visited Mum. Sandy had already alerted me that moving Mum to get dressed now seemed to cause her discomfort, so they suggested that she remained in bed. I agreed but fretted that this would mean that she'd never get up again. I'm sure they sensed that I hadn't yet fully grasped the gravity of the situation and they were right. The House Leader, Susan, gently asked me if it would help to see the foot and, when I agreed, gently peeled back the covers. Mum's swollen, discoloured foot – so purple it was almost black – looked bad. I got it now. They reassured me that it didn't seem to be giving her any pain, but they would keep checking.

I sat beside Mum's bed watching her sleep. After a while, the home manager came to see me, and we discussed what the GP had said the day before. I asked about visiting – could we visit every day now and could Aileen visit Mum in her room as well? She told me that was okay – we needed to be with our mother. As we lived in different households (and Covid rules still prevented us from mixing indoors) we could visit on separate days, but Mum would have someone with her every day. I hesitated but had one more request.

'I'm sorry to ask when you have already been so kind, but what about Ian? He's been a huge part of Mam's life and there is no way I can leave him out now. She'd want him here.'

She agreed that he could visit too. I was, and always will be, grateful for this kindness. I called Aileen and we arranged for her visit on the Wednesday, and that I would return on Thursday afternoon.

On the Thursday morning, I was delivering training online, so my phone was switched off. After the session, I realised that I had a voicemail message – one of the district nurses asking me to call her back. I quickly dialled her number. She had visited Mum that morning and she now considered her to be at end of life. My heart hit the floor – I thought we had more time with her. I raced to the care home and arranged with the manager to stay with Mum overnight.

When I reached her room, I saw that Mum's bed had been lowered down almost level with the floor. I dumped my bags in the corner of the room and sat on the carpet and curled myself up right next to where she lay, eyes closed. I took her hand – that tiny hand that I had held in so many situations – it seemed even smaller now.

'It's Helen, Mam. Helen's here,' I said, as I snuggled as close as I dared. I was afraid that the weight of my head was too heavy for her little shoulder so leaned on the pillow. We stayed like that for a while as I listened to the sound of her breathing.

'I love you, Mam,' I whispered. I thought about how many times I had said this to her over the last ten years. Probably more than in my entire life and I was glad that I had done that. Dementia had taught me to be vocal and frequent about showing my love for her. No matter what, this woman would be in no doubt that she was loved.

I have always thought that, if you have a chance, you should say all the things that you want to say to a person before they leave this life. So, on that sunny April afternoon, I thanked my mother for all she had done for me and my sisters. I thanked her for the abundance of love she gave us, the values she'd instilled in me, and the sensitive nature that I'm sure I inherited from her. I told her that all the family in Australia were thinking of her and sending their love. I nattered away, adding bits of news as I thought of them.

Later that afternoon, Ian arrived and the two of us sat quietly with her.

At around eight o'clock there was a staff shift change and Shirley, a lovely carer who had looked after Mum in the other household, popped in. She wasn't working that weekend, and I watched as she kissed Mum on the forehead and tenderly said goodbye. 'Don't worry,' I said, 'she'll see you on Monday,' – fully expecting her to still be there.

At ten o'clock it was time for Ian to go. We had agreed that he would stay until bedtime and then head off – there didn't seem any imminent change in Mum, so it made sense for just one of us to stay.

'Are you sure you are going to be okay on your own?' he asked.

'I'm fine,' I said. 'I'm exactly where I want to be – I'm with my mam.'

With the lights turned low, I settled down for the evening with a blanket over my knees watching Mum for any signs of movement and listening for changes in her breathing. I didn't want to miss a thing. Occasionally, I'd switch between the trusty recliner chair and lying on the floor next to her. I remembered being told that people could hear you, even if they are in a semi-conscious state, so I chatted to her throughout the night – then told myself off for not letting her rest.

She slept peacefully for a couple of hours at a time and then started making little groaning noises. Carers, who knew this pattern, came in every two hours, and gently asked me to leave the room while they repositioned her in the bed. Once they were done, she was quiet again. They said that she opened her eyes whenever they moved her, but of course I kept missing it. After one change, they called me back in the room quickly and I saw her eyes open – albeit briefly. I was comforted by seeing how gently the carers attended to Mum and how they watched for any changes that meant she needed pain relief. It was a peaceful night. This woman meant the world to me, and I was thankful that I could be with her.

The next morning, Aileen arrived and stayed with Mum while I went home, had a shower and a couple of hours sleep. As Aileen would be staying overnight that evening, I went back shortly after lunch and resumed my position on the floor next to Mum's bed.

That Friday afternoon will stay with me forever. I chose a Glen Campbell CD (a gift for Mum from Barbara a couple of years earlier) and, as it played, memories of us all living together flooded my thoughts. Those Sunday mornings after church with music on and Mum in the kitchen making a traditional lunch. I wished that all her girls could be with her again now. Each song seemed sadder than the one before and by the time 'Wichita Lineman' played, I was a wreck.

'D'you remember this one, Mam?' I asked our sleeping beauty, my neck now drenched with the tears that had been running down it all afternoon. Yet, it felt strangely comforting to cry for this remarkable woman who was leaving us soon. I was in no rush to pull myself together. So, as I lay on the floor, with my head next to hers, I cried some more. Occasionally, I squeezed her hand and said, 'Helen's here, Mam.' Mostly there was no response but twice she squeezed my hand back. *She's there*, I thought – and wished that for just a moment she would open her eyes.

Around mid-afternoon, Ian arrived with food and moral support. I was soothed by his presence and, as he spoke to Mum in his low gentle tones, I thought how pleased she would be that he was there. His jokes, his steady reassuring voice and his strong arms had kept both Mum and me afloat for the past ten years and it was no different now.

Aileen arrived at around eight o'clock to take over for the evening. I reminded her that we needed to contact a vicar. That afternoon, the district nurse had prompted me when she asked if Mum was religious and would she want someone from the church to visit her. *Of course she would!* I thought. Everything had happened so fast that it had completely gone out of my mind. A few days ago, I was thinking that Mum had weeks or months left, but now I knew it would only be days. Still, we had time as I was certain that she wouldn't die that day. I would make the call that night.

'Night-night, Mam,' I whispered into her ear. 'See you tomorrow.' I kissed her again and we left at 8.20 pm.

As soon as we arrived home, I called the vicar from the church where Mum and I had spent those memorable Sundays a few years earlier. He was sorry to hear the news and agreed that he would visit her the next morning. I hung up and almost immediately the phone rang again. It was Aileen.

'Helen – I think Mam's just taken her last breath. I'm not sure – someone is checking now.' I heard panic in her voice.

'Right, I'm coming back. I'll be there in five minutes, Aileen.'

Ian, who had heard only my side of the short conversation, looked at me from his armchair.

'Mam's gone,' I said, but I hoped I was wrong.

We were back in the car, down the dual carriageway, into the home and Mum's room within minutes. I looked at Aileen – she was crying. 'She's gone, Helen.' It sounded so final.

I knelt next to Mum and touched her cheek. Her body was still warm, but yes, she had died.

'Bye Mam – I love you.'

Instinctively, I felt the need to say some other goodbyes while I believed her soul was still there. I'd done this when Dad had died unexpectedly almost twenty years earlier. Barbara was in Australia and Aileen was on holiday, so I'd made a point of saying goodbye from each one of us. Now, in that cosy little bedroom, I said the name of each name of family members who weren't there and told her that they loved her and said goodbye. For a moment I thought,

I've talked her ears off for the last two days – she knows all this, but I did it anyway. When I was finished, I kissed her forehead again and held her tiny hand for the last time.

Meanwhile Aileen called Barbara. We had kept her up to date since the GP had given us the news and the district nurse announced that Mum was at end of life, so she was expecting the call. It was strange to share this significant moment over the phone in a three-way conversation – I wanted her to be there with Aileen, Ian and me. I knew that she would have given anything to have been with her mother at the end of her life but, even without Covid and international travelling bans, no one could have predicted how quickly this would happen. I was comforted that Aileen had been with Mum at the end. It didn't matter that I wasn't there for her dying breaths – Aileen was, and Mum would have known that she wasn't alone.

The care home team quietly swung into action – calling the district nurses and then the undertaker. It all happened quietly and discretely. We didn't know how long it would be before the undertaker arrived, so I suggested that Aileen go home, and that Ian and I stay with Mum until they came. She wouldn't be on her own.

After the undertakers had taken Mum's body away, we drove back home in stunned silence. I could barely believe what had happened in a matter of a few days. From the phone call from her GP on the Monday to her death at 9.10 pm on Friday 16th April was only five short days. We had lost her – not just the woman who had brought me into the world – but the person who had been a cornerstone in our lives for the past ten years. It was over. Mum was now at peace.

Chapter 30
Adored
May 2021

The next few days went by in a flurry of activity. Registering Mum's death, meetings with the undertakers, notifying family and friends. It would have felt strange in normal times but, with all the Covid restrictions, it was even more odd.

The funeral couldn't take place until three weeks later, which seemed such a long time but was the first appointment we could get. We were only allowed a handful of mourners at the crematorium, and we laboured over who we should invite. Covid rules meant that we couldn't have a wake. We couldn't meet anywhere before or after the service, weren't allowed visitors in our own homes and any indoor venues that were open had a rule of no more than six people together. *How would we do this?* Relatives who lived long distances away were happy to attend but, after considering the rules, we agreed that it was unwise. Driving for hours, attending a fifteen-minute service and not being able to have so much as a cup of tea in a café afterwards – it was a desperate situation.

Between the three of us, we managed to pull together a service that we hoped reflected our mum. We arranged for it to be streamed live so that Barbara could view it at home in Australia. The pitiful number of mourners would not reflect the number of people whose lives The Lovely Rita had touched. If it was up to me, we would have had an orchestra, a full choir, banners in the street and a chapel crammed with those who loved her. As it was, a small low-key affair was all we could manage.

Even so, on the day of the funeral, I was nervous and relieved that it had been planned for midmorning so there was no time to dwell on my sadness. Each of us had contributed something to say about our remarkable mum and, by chance, they covered various times in our lives. Aileen shared a few of her memories of Mum for the vicar to say, Barbara asked Ian to read out her eulogy and I was determined that I was going to say something to honour her. I didn't want to shy away from her experience with dementia and wanted to speak about what she had given us in those years, despite her difficulties. She (and ironically the disease) had taught me so much about love and relationships that I didn't want her last years to be remembered only with sadness.

Helen's Eulogy for her Mam

Our mam touched so many people's lives over the years and everyone has special memories of The Lovely Rita. Today, I would like to share my memories of Mam from the last ten years or so.

Despite the difficulties that living with dementia brought her, Mam still brought love and joy into our lives. Her sweet nature and gentle ways made it easy for people to love her. Friends – old and new, carers and other health professionals – all took Rita to their hearts and have a story to tell of her. Everyone here today will know at least one of her funny sayings or have heard her quick wit.

Mam was the ultimate in showing gratitude and living in the moment. Even her fortnightly appointment at the foot clinic would become a special outing in the car, with an opportunity for a singalong and a packet of Quavers for the return journey. She was happy with even the smallest things.

Then there were the Sunday Adventures that Mam, Ian and I had for many years. A visit to a cafe at the coast, the Rising Sun country park, or to a garden centre – would all end up with a cup of tea and a scone. Much later, when getting in and out of the car was too much of a chore, we introduced her to the McDonald's Drive Thru for a hot chocolate or McFlurry Ice Cream. She loved the experience. We'd then go to the lake in Killingworth and watch the swans or, as Mam would say, 'the ducks in the watter'. I like to think that those days out brought Mam happiness, but boy, did she reward us with so much love and fun in return.

Mam was always very creative. She wrote many verses and poems – often for friends who had suffered a loss. So, it seems right that one of her poems is in the Order of Service today. Her love for painting, all things in nature and friendships did not diminish in the latter years and you could always find something to interest her. She was known for her neat curly hair, her smart clothes and jewellery, and I thank every carer who took the time to help mum preserve her glamorous look. Who knew that she'd even become a model at eighty-seven?

*Dementia brought us close and although I would wish the disease away – I am grateful for every minute I had with her. She was never in the background of our lives – she was front and centre. **She was adored.** It was in these years, that Mam unwittingly taught us an important part of every relationship. That is: It is not just about what you do – it is how you make me feel. This will stay with me forever, Mam.*

I will never forget the joy of seeing her beautiful smile as I walked into the room. That smile filled my heart with love. After each visit, she would give me a gentle wave and say 'bye pet' – again melting my heart.

So now it is time for us to say goodbye to her, but I know she would want each one of us to be happy and live well. Later you will see some photos of Rita in the last few years that show her loving, funny, playful personality. Please remember her like that – as we will. Our mam – The Lovely Rita.

*****

Years before, I had said that when Mum eventually died, we wouldn't have the usual photo of our demure mum on the top of the coffin for mourners to see. I wanted a slide show of photos showing the funny faces she pulled over the years – making us all laugh. Now that the time had come, I wasn't sure that I would get my wish. When I mentioned it at the undertaker's office, Aileen was horrified but, after a bit more discussion (and checking the photos), both sisters eventually agreed. So, at the end of the funeral service, to the sound of Nat King Cole's 'Unforgettable', the tiny group of mourners saw a slideshow of Rita pulling her countless funny faces. The last photo: waving goodbye.

Rita's Poem

There is a lovely legend, that's still believed today,
that God created mothers in a very special way.
He took a dash of wisdom to this he added love,
and mixed in all the kindness he could find from up above.
And when He was all finished, he sent them from the skies,
today we call them mothers, but they're angels in disguise.

Peace is yours. Memories are ours.
Rita Johns (Date unknown)

*****

December 2022

After more than a year without Mum, I miss her every day and know that I will miss her for ever. I miss seeing her radiant smile, the smell of her perfume (always Aromatics) and holding her tiny hand. I miss buying the jewellery sets that she adored and other 'treasures' that I delighted in finding to keep her active and stimulated. But I am glad it is over – for her and for us.

For Mum, living with dementia was tough, but the trauma of the disease was not the whole story. The care home environment, her relationship with carers and her family, and how she spent her day, all determined whether she lived well with dementia – or not. I did not know that when we started out, but I know it now.

My mother's experience of care – and my observation of it – exposed me and my family to the highs and lows of a system that is complicated and often felt broken. I met many kind, hardworking and caring people who touched Mum's life in a positive way. I am grateful for them and thank them for everything they did. I also met others who do not deserve the same praise, and I am perplexed as to how this can exist in a modern world of dementia care.

I am sad that the plans that we made for a carefree summer in Mum's new home never came to fruition. I feel a hole deep in my stomach when I think about the Covid year (from February 2020) that stopped me from spending cherished time with her as I'd done in the years before. Maybe the rate of her decline would still have been the same – although I don't think so – but, even if it had, I would have been by her side. I would have nurtured her through those final stages of dementia and stayed close to her until the very end. Instead, it is the care staff who have those memories of the occasional words she uttered, the cute smile that lit up her face, and her loving gaze upon them. I am grateful that they were there to look after her so well, but envious that they saw what I was forbidden to experience when she was locked away from me and my sisters. I am not alone in this feeling – thousands of people missed the opportunity of being with their loved ones in their last days. I know that I was fortunate to have had our visits properly restored in March 2021, just before she finally left us.

I've had lots of time to reflect on the (almost) ten years during which dementia and the care home system dominated our lives, and my feelings have mellowed somewhat. That is, until I read current reports about some new injustice in the care system: relatives still blocked from visiting, failings in services that leave relatives bereft; or I overhear a cliché about care staff or relatives. Then I return to the fierce side of Helen that wants to scream, 'Something has got to change!'

In this book, I have tried to convey how Mum felt and how that made me feel – which in turn, drove my actions. Those years were excruciatingly tough, but it was a privilege to care for my beautiful mother. Dementia brought us close and fostered in me a deep love for her that I previously never knew existed. Her wellbeing became my priority – day in and day out. The experience has changed me. It has changed how I view social care in general and my opinion on how we care for those living with dementia. It has changed my career and the values I hold dear. For several years now, I have devoted my working life to various aspects of social care – and that experience has consolidated my view: *there has to be a better way for us to provide authentic and compassionate care.*

Part 4

A Better Way for All of Us

Introduction

In a world where the budget for social care is always under pressure, there are no easy fixes. With staff shortages and other demands on the system, it would be madness if the valuable resource of relatives and friends was not harnessed and used as 'partners in care'. If things are to get better for those living with dementia, then relatives and care teams need to work together to support their wellbeing.

An equal and mutually respectful relationship, between those who have known the person before they 'became' a resident and those who take on the responsibility of more formal care, *can* be achieved. But, if that is to happen, we need to dispel some of the common myths that I have heard over the years. They have grown and developed so much in care home folklore that they can often be deemed as fact. From my personal and professional experience – I would like to offer an alternative perspective.

Myth 1: All relatives feel guilty

The common message is that relatives feel guilty about 'putting' their loved one in a care home and it is because of that guilt that they nit-pick about the care. I have heard this numerous times, particularly when carers talk casually about relatives. I am not able to speak for other relatives, but I would like to share my take on this.

I never felt guilt about making the decision that Mum needed to live in a care home. The decision was made because she needed 24-hour care that neither I nor my sisters were able to provide. Had

Mum been less anxious, perhaps we could have found a way, but the urgent and frightening manifestation of dementia meant that she needed professional help immediately. Would I have felt guilty seeking an appropriate environment for any of her other health conditions? No – so why would I for *this* type of care?

What I did feel, though, was an overwhelming sense of sadness, frustration and anger that she wasn't fully helped to thrive in that environment. I wanted the care home and dementia care to be better.

My suggestion: Relatives do not always feel guilty, but they DO want good care outcomes for their loved ones.

Myth 2: Relatives are either too controlling or simply 'dump' their loved ones

Again, casual conversations I've heard indicate a view held by some care staff that relatives fall into one of the following categories: (a) they are overcontrolling and reluctant to let the carers do their job; or (b) they have 'dumped' their loved ones and walked away from them.

In my experience, families are eternally grateful for any release from the responsibilities of care duties that having a person moving into a care home brings. However, having often had that responsibility for a long time, they do not want to see a dip in the quality of their loved one's care. They have learnt to be vigilant about their relative's health, so it is natural for them to adopt that same approach to the handover of care. The fact that their loved one is now in a care home does not make that feeling of responsibility for their health and wellbeing fade.

Others, for various reasons, do not want to know too much detail about the day-to-day care – but still want their loved one to be well looked-after. Either way, relatives do not want to be overlooked or ignored but they do appreciate being informed and consulted.

In a bid to fit in with the home, relatives often overlook the small infringements regarding a person's wellbeing and only react when breaches increase to an unacceptable level.

My suggestion: Most often relatives want to work as a partner in care with care teams.

Myth 3: Everything is down to the dementia.

For so many problems that Mum (and others) faced, carers were keen to write them off as a symptom of dementia. This was not always the case. Yes, dementia often exacerbated the confusion around an issue or a misinterpretation of events. However, for Mum, the environment she lived in, the people around her and the things that were said and done played a bigger part.

I saw instances where people supported her to live well. I saw others who either unwittingly confused her more or casually undermined her – both of which increased her disability.

My suggestion: Residents react appropriately for the position they find themselves in. Address the source of their feelings and you can often address the problem effectively.

Myth 4: There isn't a way to live well with dementia.

Similar to the above point, assumptions are often made about the outlook for a person living with dementia. When Mum was first diagnosed, I felt that her days of happiness were at an end. However, what I found was that there were ways for us to live in the moment with Mum and, when we did that, she enjoyed herself or felt calm. Over time, we found different ways to introduce happy times for

Mum and we tried to stitch those times together to form happy hours and days.

My suggestion: Let us disregard the above assumptions and open our mind to what is possible. There are ways to support a person to live well with the disease – we just have to look for them.

Myth 5: What you say really isn't important for those who have memory problems – generally they can't understand.

I sometimes heard careless language in care homes that made me wince. Examples that spring to mind include:

- A carer, not knowing the resident's name and trying to describe them to a colleague, saying, 'Thingy has lost her purse. *It's the one* who gets her hair done.'

- Talking about a resident as if they were not in the room.

- Discussing a resident's care within earshot of other residents.

- Scolding a resident when they didn't understand they needed to stay in their room when poorly. 'Okay – then let's see what happens when you make everyone else ill!'

I felt frustrated in homes where the otherwise kind, well-intentioned care staff would fall into these bad habits. In some cases, homes did the 'window-dressing' about treating people with respect and dignity but didn't follow this up with action to embed it within the culture of the home.

My suggestion: The message that I discovered from the Scottish Care Inspectorate initiative (mentioned in chapter 22) is so important:

'It's not just what you do ... it's how you make me feel.'

I've heard expressions such as 'Nobody can make you feel bad without your permission' or similar sentiments and generally I would agree with this. However, when it comes to dementia – when we rely on our feelings most – I view things differently.

How a person feels becomes even more important as the other cognitive functions decline. People living with dementia will sense a disrespectful tone, will feel the lack of warmth in a person's voice and will feel vulnerable because of it.

Remember this sentiment and it will help guide you to do and say the right thing.

A better way for all of us: relatives and care teams

When I first decided to write this book, I thought: *how about I put some general tips and hints at the end?* Then, I remembered the hundreds of conversations I'd had with Debbie about living in Daughterville. As professionals who worked in the sector, we kept asking ourselves, 'What can be done to change things?' Whenever one of us had an idea, the other would say something like, 'I know, but don't the local authority contracts cover that?' or 'Yes – but the inspectors look at that bit.' We realised that the problem was the *gap* between what was:

(a) intended by the care home;

(b) expected by the contracting bodies and inspectorates; and

(c) actually experienced by the person on the receiving end.

In such a heavily regulated sector, there is no shortage of contracts, standards and manuals to guide the practice but there is a shortage of scrutiny on how care feels from the resident's perspective. Not just on the week of an audit or inspection, but over an extended period.

For me, it often felt like a case of *The Emperor's New Clothes*, where everyone seemed to believe that things were working or feared pointing out the obvious: that care home life, in many instances, wasn't a good experience.

Therefore, there is little merit in me suggesting tips that say, 'The care home should do …' – because the care home brochure and website will, no doubt, say that this already happens.

So, what advice *would* I give to someone choosing a care home? What would I say to those in the sector *who truly want to change?* Here is a collection of suggestions that might help someone who finds themselves in the same position that we were in ten years ago. I also share some ideas of things that would have made us feel supported by the care team.

The following should not be taken as professional advice – it is simply what worked for us. To be more accurate, it is what *could have worked* if it had been implemented fully! Nevertheless, I share it here as you may find some of the ideas helpful.

I have divided my thoughts into the following key areas:

- finding a care home and the first four weeks of care

- dealing consistently with difficult questions/distressed behaviour

- focussing on how a person spends their day

- when things go wrong.

Finding a care home and the first four weeks of care

Relatives and Friends

- Visit as many care homes as you can, as early as you can. Do it before you end up, as we did, in a crisis situation. Visit at different times of day so that you can observe the atmosphere at different times.

- Ask what I now consider to be one of the most important questions in selecting a home: **'How will my mum [dad, partner, friend] spend their day?'** This will give you an indication of how the home supports residents to retain their wellbeing.

- Ask how the care home finds out about the resident's preferences and how families can share information with the staff team.

- Ask how often the care will be reviewed and if relatives can be involved in this meeting. This will set up a regular way to communicate with the home management.

- Look carefully at what is going on around you during your visits? **Do residents look *contented and well cared for*? How do staff engage with them?**

Once you have selected a home:

- **Share the information** you have about your relative's life history, personality, preferences and abilities in written form – and reinforce it verbally.

- **Ask questions about the home** and gather information in the same way you would in a new job. Find out the practical stuff that goes beyond what's in the glossy brochures, for example:

'How often are the rooms cleaned?' or 'Where should I put the dirty laundry?'

Care Home Managers/Carers

- **Encourage relatives** to share what they know about the person coming to live in the home and ensure that this is recorded in the care plan.

- Managers – allow care staff time to read and digest any **Life History material** and ensure they understand that a key part of their role is to *get to know the person* they are caring for.

- **Acknowledge the resident's prior life experience** and recognise that the resident and the relative have a bond that predates your inclusion in the caring partnership.

- **Respect the relative's existing knowledge** and valuable insight – use it to help support the resident. They have probably already been managing their relative's care for several years before they came to live in your care home.

- Provide new residents and their families with a **good, solid induction** to the home. Give them enough information to make themselves comfortable and help them to not commit any 'newbie' gaffes.

- **Empower and train your staff** to deal with a flood of questions in the beginning. Encourage relatives to ask any little thing that may be playing on their mind. Do this early and you will make them feel confident and comfortable in your home.

- Create a feeling of being **'in this together'** with relatives. It is far preferable to a **'them and us'** situation, which makes everyone feel tense.

- The term, 'My door is always open', is often used by managers. Make sure you mean it and that residents and relatives *feel* that this is the case.

Dealing consistently with difficult questions/ distressed behaviours

Relatives and Friends

- As part of the 'getting-to-know-you' process, agree on what are the likely questions that will need answering (e.g. 'Where's my husband?' – especially if deceased).

- **Agree on a form of words** that stays as near to the truth as possible without risking upsetting the person repeatedly.

- Be consistent with the message. If one relative says, 'Dad is on holiday' and another says, 'He's at work and will be in at 5 pm', this will only confuse the person more.

- Whatever is said, make sure that the response:

  ◦ Acknowledges the feeling ('You must be worried about [X]').

  ◦ Responds to the question ('I haven't heard from …').

  ◦ Opens up an opportunity to discuss the person ('Look at this photo of [X]').

- I learnt that most distressed behaviour comes from an **'unmet need'**. Work with the home and try to identify that need. If necessary, ask if outside help is available.

Care Home Managers/Carers

- Work with the family to agree **the form of words** that could be used to respond to difficult questions.

- Reassure families and explain how you will honour the resident by using therapeutic lies (if that is your approach) only when necessary and **in a consistent way**.

- Agree how you will keep the family informed, and how regularly. They will appreciate your honesty.

Focussing on how a person spends their day

Relatives and Friends

- It is important that the person who goes to live in a care home can keep doing the things that have been part of their life. It can be easy to give up and stop doing things when cognitive decline makes them difficult. Getting support from others can help (for example, in our case friends made it possible for Mum to continue to go to church for a while).

- If you know your loved one **enjoys a particular hobby** (e.g. knitting), make sure you take any equipment into the home and help them to continue to do the things that make them feel like themselves. Do not be put off. Find a way to adapt things to suit the person as they are now.

- Enjoy the **uneventful but precious moments** with your loved one. There were moments when, despite the worries, I felt the sheer joy of just sitting next to my beautiful mum. Sometimes that is enough for both of you.

- Having a strong support team of friends and relatives who can visit a loved one in a care home is beneficial as it helps them to stay connected to their lives and shares the caring responsibilities.

- If you find that the home doesn't have much going on in the way of meaningful activity – be persistent with your requests. **Keep asking**, 'What activities are available today?' and 'What is there for my mum [dad, partner, friend] to do this week?'

- Seeing your loved one, and others, living in a care home can be daunting. The sights and sounds can, at first, be unnerving and it may be tempting to stay away. Try to stick with it, for the greater good of your loved one. It gets easier and, as in my case, you may grow to like or even love fellow residents.

Care Home Managers/Carers

- Ask yourself regularly, 'How do residents spend their day?' and 'Is this how they would choose to spend their time?' **Be honest with your responses**. If you think living in your care home must be boring – you are probably right.

- If you have activity coordinators – check that the activity programme truly reflects the preferences of the current resident population. It is easy to fall into the trap of providing an activity programme of bingo, singalongs and movie nights – just because you think that's what people might like. Check what people say they enjoy, and build your programme around that.

- Encourage and support relatives and friends to be an **integral part of your home,** rather than just 'visitors'. Encourage them to join in with activities and events, or help them find a way to adapt activities during their visits. Ask for volunteers to host sessions – you will be using people's skills to enhance your home.

- **Provide private areas** where people can sit quietly and have a conversation. Nothing is more off-putting for a visitor than having to shout over a noisy TV in the lounge.

When things go wrong

Relatives and Friends

Be prepared that even when you are justifiably, politely and patiently pointing out what has gone wrong, the care home manager may not take this as a helpful intervention. There are ways, however, to prevent this tricky situation from becoming worse.

- **Raise your concerns as soon as possible** after the event/incident has happened. Delaying it will not help. Be precise about what happened and when it happened.

- Tell the manager (politely) how it made you feel and how you believe it makes your loved one feel. **Focus on the impact** it has on the resident rather than whether a task was done or not done. For example, I emphasised that leaving Mum's waist slip off made her feel uncomfortable (it did) – not that it irritated me (it did!).

- If something happens repeatedly, **make notes** so that you can show evidence of a pattern.

- When times are tough it can be difficult to find anything positive to say – I found the following helpful:

  ○ Start with what has worked well (even if it is only a tiny part).

  ○ Move on to what needs to be improved.

  ○ Respectfully ask what they will do to make sure the same thing doesn't happen again (this is the most important step).

- **If necessary, formalise** things by using the organisation's complaints process.

Care Home Managers/Carers

- Nothing is more frustrating than seeing something go wrong and no one having the confidence to tackle it. If something goes wrong, please give relatives the reassurance they need by:

  ○ Acknowledging that it happened.

  ○ Identifying why it happened and what went wrong.

  ○ Having something in place that will stop the same thing from happening again.

  ○ Once you have done the above, checking that it is not continuing to happen.

- Relatives will respect a manager **who is visible** and knows what is happening around their home. If you aren't regularly in the lounges, talking to residents and staff, you won't see what relatives see every day.

- Poor communication is often the source of problems. If you have good handover techniques and other communication tools, you can alleviate many problems.

- When you are on the 'receiving end' of a negative comment about care from relatives or friends, understand that their primary concern is for their loved one. That stern look or that abrupt tone may stem from overwhelming fear and worry. **Put yourself in their position** and find a way to work together to resolve issues.

These suggestions cover some of the recurring themes that arose for me when Mum lived in a care home. There are many organisations who can provide good, professionally researched advice and guidance to add to the above suggestions. I have listed some of these in the *References* section of this book.

I wish you courage and I wish you well in your care home journey.

Helen

x .

References

Alzheimer's Society - Information about dementia, fact sheets, advice etc.
https://www.alzheimers.org.uk/

Daily Sparkle - Reminiscence newspaper and quality resources for Activity Professionals.
https://www.dailysparkle.co.uk/

Dementia Friends - An Alzheimer's Society initiative to change people's perceptions of dementia.
https://www.dementiafriends.org.uk/

Healthwatch - An independent health and social care champion.
https://www.healthwatch.co.uk/

NAPA - Information, advice and support on all issues relating to activity, arts and engagement)
https://napa-activities.co.uk/

Make Every Moment Count - A Scottish Care Inspectorate initiative. *The five messages are reproduced in chapter 22 with the kind permission of the Care Inspectorate.*
https://hub.careinspectorate.com/media/3791/make-every-moment-count-a-guide-for-everyday-living.pdf

The Relatives & Residents Association - The national charity for older people needing care and the relatives and friends who help them cope.
https://www.relres.org/

Rights For Residents - A campaign to end the restrictions to visiting loved ones in care homes.
https://www.rightsforresidents.co.uk/

The Bookcase Analogy – You Tube. A non-scientific explanation of how memory works.

Inspectorates Governing Care Homes
The following organisations are the regulators of adult social care in the relevant countries. Their websites include reports on care homes and other resources which you may find useful.

England
Care Quality Commission (CQC)
https://www.cqc.org.uk/

Scotland
The Care Inspectorate
https://www.careinspectorate.com/

Wales
Care Inspectorate Wales
https://www.careinspectorate.wales/

Northern Ireland
The Regulation and Quality Improvement Authority (RQIA)
https://www.rqia.org.uk/

Republic of Ireland
The Health Information and Quality Authority (HIQA)
https://www.hiqa.ie/

About the Author

Helen Johns lives in North East England with husband Ian. Her career (unwittingly) divided itself into 10-year chunks. The first chunk was in fashion retail, including a stint with Selfridges in London. The next decade was dedicated to post-16 special needs education for a national training company. It was here that she honed her excellent training skills. She then established her own training & consultancy service and for the next 10 years worked on large national education reform projects. In 2012 everything changed. Helen's Mum was diagnosed with dementia. Moved by the vulnerabilities of those living with the disease, Helen felt compelled to switch her focus to training within Health & Social care. This world of dementia care and meaningful activity has been her passion for the last 10 years.

Follow her on social media.

Website www.hmjconsultancy.co.uk
Facebook https://facebook.com/hmjauthor
Twitter: https://twitter.com/DementiaReThink
Email: helen@hmjconsultancy.co.uk

Printed in Great Britain
by Amazon

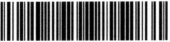

44139102R00169